Back In The Swirl:
Coping With Meniere's Vertigo, Migraines, Chronic Depression and Baffled Doctors

MERCEDES KIM-CABRERA

ISBN: 978-1-4669-9495-9 (sc)
ISBN: 978-1-4669-9497-3 (hc)
ISBN: 978-1-4669-9496-6 (e)

Library of Congress Control Number: 2013909402

Trafford rev. 08/23/2013

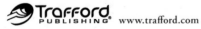 www.trafford.com

North America & international
toll-free: 1 888 232 4444 (USA & Canada)
fax: 812 355 4082

CONTENTS

To Jesus, Mary and Michael.
To Blanca, Olga, Mary and Marlene.
To my children.

PROLOGUE

Mrs. Russell and I wash and watch. Simultaneously. We wash a huge load of microscope glass slides used by the Microbiology lab students the prior day. We lather, scrub, scrape and rinse in a repetitive motion. All the while we watch Bo and Hope full-fledged, passionate romance in *Days Of Our Lives.* Mrs. Russell is in charge of the Undergraduate Microbiology Laboratory situated at the Arts and Science Building. It is my last semester at the University of Miami, my alma mater. I truly do not care that much for the soap opera but Mrs. Russell has gotten me hooked up on it. She has been my boss for the past two years. I am an undergraduate student on a scholarship. My part-time job at the lab allows me to earn funds to supplement my financial aid package. We submerge our slides in a big plastic bucket that contains detergent. Soap and soap. Pun intended.

It is year 1983. I gaze at the tiny screen of the mini TV set sitting on the Formica counter across our metal chairs. Mrs. Russell, an American of Irish descent, has tended to the UM Microbiology lab for over thirty ears. It is her now her turn to retire to her family, dogs and cats and her fabulous house nestled in the old, charming city of Coral Gables. She has earned it.

I am in my last semester. I am about to receive my Bachelor's in Microbiology and Immunology. We both are feisty today. We have so much to celebrate. Mrs. Russell is looking forward to a well-deserved life of leisure. I am looking forward to a new full-time employment in my career field, entering graduate school, marriage and eventually a family to call my own.

It is my last day of work. I am done. I dry the last slide, place it carefully in its cardboard box and grab my colorful fringed book bag. Mrs. Russell wrinkled face brims a big smile. Her intense blue eyes look at me with delight. Her arms extend open wide. She embraces me, pats my back and slides a white envelope into my right hand.

"What's this?" I say with a quizzical look on my face.

"Ah. Here is the key to opening your golden door. This is a recommendation letter for you. Take her to Dr. Violet Aschkinks in the Transplant department. She will help you to get your first full-time job after graduation. Violet is a good, old friend of mine. She is in charge of the Kidney Transplantation Unit. You'll be in great hands. Good luck sweetie. You deserve it!"

Her eyes beam with the proudness of a mother who finally sees her hard work of years rewarded in her offspring's college degree. And why not? Ms. Russell has been my mentor for two years. She has been my steadfast guide in the difficult world of courses selections, in the choosing of the most flexible professors in the Microbiology department, she has shown me the ropes, the ABC's of a microbiology laboratory, she might have thrown two or three romantic tips regarding my amorous relationship with my boyfriend, and finally, she has been a very patient and encouraging instructor of her native language.

As a "Cuban refugee" living in the States for only two years, it has not been short of a challenge to maneuver around the sophisticated, exclusively scientific vocabulary of my PH.D's educators and my shortcomings regarding the most widely used language in the world. Ms. Russell has been an invaluable help! I blow her a kiss with my hands and I fly down the old-grayish concrete stairs of the Arts and Science building. I fly into my new world of financial freedom, achieved dreams, and the satisfaction that hard work always pays. I have done it. I have prevailed. My flight abruptly stops when I land into my fiancee's strong, muscular arms and I melt into his hazel eyes and press my lips against his savoring my triumph. My baby has been eagerly waiting for me to celebrate my last school day. I envision our future path, marriage, a house, a successful career, and eventually children. What else can I ask for? I don't want my fly ever to end.

Forward three months later, half of the deal is sealed. The other half is irretrievably broken. I have landed my starter dream job at the Transplant unit in my alma mater. My baby and I on the other hand, are separated. We have parted away (my own decision) and now I totally regret it. I can only pray for the miracle of forgiveness. And while I am anxiously waiting for it (my miracle) I am ecstatic about my new surroundings. I work full-time at both a clinical and a research lab at the Transplant unit. I am moving up steadily on my laboratory certifications and planning my upcoming graduate school entrance exam. My life is still full, adventurous and the future is brighter than ever. I am secretly dreaming, planning and expecting. Until the day all hell breaks loose and my life starts spinning out of control. Literally. Pun intended.

Alina, a laboratory colleague, tucks at my lab coat and nudges me gently towards the hall. I quickly take it off and wash my hands thoroughly. Sue and Kathy, another two young lab co-workers, join us and amid laughter and lively chatting we head off to the nearest elevator. By the time we reach the cafeteria entrance I feel a sudden wave of heat burning my face. I leave out a quiet sigh as unsuccessfully try to reach for the door knob. Everything becomes blurry in front of me; I close my eyes, lose control and inevitably fall down to the floor with a hard thump. My unconsciousness lasts only for a few minutes. My vital signs are checked by my friends and when nothing is out of the ordinary, I get up and proceed to eat our lunch. The rest of the afternoon glides easily into the fasts-paced routines of my work. I wrap up the day and leave work feeling perfectly normal.

I have just reunited with my lost love and we are barely starting anew when I am seized by an unexpected fall and loss of consciousness while at work. This is the only time I would pass out. From there on, my unconsciousness is replaced by a new array of symptoms. In the subsequent weeks and months, my world *spins* completely out of control. Vertigo, unrelenting upchucking, loss of balance, fatigue and a disturbing fullness sensation and continuous ringing in my ears are my increasingly steadfast companions.

For the next three years my life is reduced to the enclosing four walls of my room in my tiny apartment. I spend not one, or two, but three years homebound. I just cling to my misery, bedridden, continuously vomiting; either gyrating along with my room or my room spinning vertiginously around me.

I had survived episodic, paternal abuse in my childhood, broken family bonds generated by exile in my adolescence, a perilous sea voyage from Cuba but nothing has prepared me for the inferno I am facing now. It would take three years of my young life, numerous clueless, baffled doctors, the loss of my amazingly, challenging job, the abandonment of most of my friends, three failed attempted suicides and finally, a totally unexpected trip to Emory Hospital in Atlanta and the return to the roots of my Catholic faith before a diagnosis is finally pronounced—Meniere's disease. Three years before a new treatment eliminates my incapacitating, devastating symptoms. Three whole years before my vertigo subsides. I am finally confident to look ahead to the future I have forged in my mind.

For the next sixteen years my dreams are fulfilled. I am back in the medicine field. I have a husband, a career, and three beautiful, healthy Asian children. No, I did not adopt. My husband is of Asian descent. Who would have thought? More importantly, I have reconnected to the God who was introduced to me in my infant years by my aunt and uncle. We now have a solid, interactive, vivid relationship based on a daily communication and the absolute, irrefutable proof of His unconditional love. I need no more.

November 2007. It is my forty sixth birthday anniversary. My husband, I, and our children are visiting with my old, closest friend from my youth, Elizabeth. Eli and I go back from our early adolescence in our country. We hit it off from the first time we met in eighth grade. We have been inseparable from the day we met. Although we are in the month of November, Miami hot climate year-round makes it very pleasant to take a dip in a swimming pool. We are sitting in Eli's Spanish-tile covered backyard terrace savoring the lazy Sunday afternoon. I am watching the kids Eli's and mine splashing in the pool, running around it, enjoying another care-free day of their young lives. I take a sip from my chilled, pink lemonade beverage. I drag a puff of my Virginia slim. Just then, I feel it. The ringing, the buzzing, the fullness in my ears and the strange feeling that overtakes my whole body; the old, too familiar malaise that precedes the attack. It is the crisis that would drastically change my life once again.

I load myself with Xanax and anti-nausea pills. I lie down in Eli's mom bed. I don't dare to move at all except to vomit the delicious meal I had savored a while ago. It takes what it seems forever before the pharmaceuticals render me motionless and sound asleep. A last thought pounds my mind. *After sixteen years of remission, all of your confidence about being symptom-free, all the reassurance that you have conquered and prevailed you are back to being the poor-disabled-afflicted by relentless vertigo Mercy.*

Mercy you are back, Back in the Swirl of . . . Meniere.

As my world tumbles down like years ago, my predicament intensifies as if that is even possible. Nothing could break the hold Meniere has over my life. I have transcended the most feared complication of my illness. I used to have one ear affected by Meniere. Now, both of my ears are compromised. I have Bilateral Meniere, the most challenging medical scenario an ENT doctor can encounter in the realm of Meniere. Having both ears impacted by Meniere makes it impossible for me to have any surgical or any other aggressive treatment usually reserved for the most desperate cases of vertigo. When both ears are taken by Meniere, these treatments are off-limits. Permanent loss of balance is a real complication of last recourse Meniere treatments. There is just not a "good ear" left to compensate for the balance loss. To compound the problem, I have been diagnosed with chronic depression since year 2000. I have to contend with two extremely debilitating conditions from now on. I reach the end of the rope.

I am transfixed with the battle ahead of me. Hismanal (Astemizole), the drug that brought my vertigo to a halt some long years ago, is no longer available. It has been banned by the FDA as the result of severe heart complications, including fatality cases. For the next two years the macabre cycle is back. I hug the toilet, I vomit for twenty hours continuously, I lose my balance, I am dizzy, I can't walk, I load my body with anti-vertigo meds, I am exhausted. I fall asleep. I can't do anything. I have no life. My three children have to fend for themselves, survive on their own while their father work long hours and mommy is alive but so ill that she literally lives in her bed. The caring, devoted mother of the past ceases to exist. How do you explain to three young children that their mother lies motionless in bed for years, victim of an illness that is not terminal as their deceased uncle's cancer but equally crippling? You cannot. The kids can't grasp this new reality. Fortunately, compassionate souls reach out to my family. I have to let go of all expectations.

One day my boy enters my room after a long day spent at school. His usually bright, caramel-colored eyes reflect all the melancholy and preoccupation that invades him.

"Mom, how do you do it? If I were you I would have jumped off the balcony long ago."

I am perplexed, appalled at his audacious statement. We live on a fifth floor, jumping off means a certain death. Why do I put up with all this misery?

"Because of you my son, because of your sisters, because a captain does not abandon his ship strayed into perilous waters. Neither does a mother abandon her children." I barely whisper in reply. I tentatively extend my hand from under my cover and stroke his dark hair. I close my eyes and go back to the fog that envelops me constantly. I can't surrender. I have come so far now just to give up. It is not in my nature.

My children are the main force that propels me into a new quest. I need a huge break, a miracle. It arrives one day when a mother from my girls' school tells me all about her own father's experience at the Silverstein Institute in Sarasota. Her dad, a Meniere veteran, had endured intractable vertigo for quite a while when he met Dr. Herbert Silverstein, the founder of the Institute. Dr. Silverstein performed an operation that cured his vertigo completely. After two years of unabatedly vertigo, I visit the Institute myself. Although my Meniere presents itself as the worst type to be successfully treated because both ears are affected by the illness, disqualifying me from more aggressive treatments such as surgery, Dr. Silverstein prescribes a new medication for my condition.

The trip to Sarasota marks the end of my marriage of almost twenty years. My husband and I take a fork on the road. I am devastated. I am on my own, disabled and still very ill. Yet, little by little in the course of the following months I start to see a gradual improvement. As soon as my divorce is finalized, I move on my own. New, unforeseeable challenges await me in my new life. Stress renders me with chronic asthma; the newest obstacle on my path to recovery. Interestingly enough, in spite of my recently diagnosed asthma, my migraines, my depression, my congenital leg condition and Meniere, vertigo begin to subside. Is Dr. Silverstein one-of-a-kind, progressive treatment dramatically enhancing the quality of my life? Yes, it is. It takes a few months for the new medication to become effective but my walker becomes a thing of the past. Am I able to do all the activities most people take for granted and that I have been deprived from for so long? Yes, I do. Little by little, I show my face back in the condominium gym, I bask in the sun by the pool, I swim, I read, I write, I cook, I drive, I can sit down in my living room and watch TV! I get to worship at my temple and most importantly, I am actively present in my children's lives again. I am out of the *Swirl*.

I don't deceive myself. Meniere has no cure. Symptoms flare up from time to time. I will always have to be cautious and keep safe boundaries to avoid a major crisis. Yet, I am forever indebted to Dr. Silverstein. Those who are affected by Meniere know that vertigo render us, its victims, in a perpetual, pathetic state with no end on sight. Meniere robs us of all desire to keep on struggling. It leaves us in utter despair, begging for an end to our miserable lives. I am blessed beyond words. I have prevailed. I have defeated the beast. Once again.

A successful vertigo treatment breathes a new life into my body and soul. There are simply no words to describe my gratitude to my family, friends who stand by me, my doctors and their expertise and finally to our God who looks down upon us with compassionate love. If my story inspires other people to come up higher, better, stronger from an epic battle against Meniere, depression or any other chronic medical condition, my journey has not been in vain. I have fulfilled my purpose in life.

INTRODUCTION

A aaah! The Starry Night. Beautiful, famous, invaluable. Who is not acquainted with this masterpiece painting and his deeply disturbed, unfortunate creator, Vincent van Gogh? Although, it was not documented during his lifetime it has been determined many years later, that van Gogh suffered from an incurable, relentless, devilish illness; Meniere's disease.

Commonly called "glaucoma of the inner ear," Meniere's disease is a chronic illness that often affects individuals in the prime of life. It is characterized by episodes of severe vertigo, loss of balance, tinnitus (ringing in the ears), nausea, vomiting and progressive hearing loss.

The National Institutes of Health estimates that about 615,000 people in the United States have Meniere's. Approximately 450,000 new cases are diagnosed annually in the country. Meniere's symptoms, especially vertigo can wreak havoc in affected patient's lives. The disease has a very serious psychosocial impact in its victims and their families. In the Quality of Wellbeing Scale, a scientific study, it is stated that Meniere's sufferers are the most severely impaired non hospitalized patients studied so far. The quality of life of a Meniere's patient is comparable to that of a Cancer or Aids patient. When having acute attacks, the Quality of Wellbeing is closer to a non-institutionalized Cancer or Aids victim . . . six days before death!

It is well documented that Meniere's sufferers fall prey to depression in alarming numbers due to their almost non-existing quality of life. In my own case, both illnesses are concomitantly present. Mental disorders are very common in the United States and internationally. Globally, the percentage of people with psychiatric disorders is growing faster than those of heart disease. The present worldwide state of economic turmoil is increasing those numbers exponentially. An estimated 22% of Americans ages 18 and older (about 1 in 5 adults) suffer from a mental condition; that's approximately 44 million people. The direct costs of mental health illness services in the United States is over $70 billion. The indirect costs are over 78 billion. The latter refers to lost productivity at the workplace, school, and home due to premature disability and death. Over 90% of suicides are committed by people who suffer from a mental illness. These staggering figures have been the inspiration to write about my vast personal experience dealing with both health conditions.

Van Gogh was so miserable in his affliction that in an extremely radical measure he severed his left ear in attempt to alleviate his highly disturbing Meniere's symptoms. Meniere compounded with other illnesses, among them a severe mental condition, finally claimed the life of the painter in his late thirties at his own hand.

My story's priority is to help Meniere's and depression sufferers to resort to less drastic measures to cope with these co-occurring illnesses, counteract their unpredictability and guide them to regain control of their live; allowing to experience their God giving right to a fulfilling, rich and active life as possible. It provides useful, unique tools and guides to overcome the turbulence and chaos in those afflicted by Meniere and chronic depression (compounded by migraines). It is my most fervent desire that my story serves as an inspiration to all patients affected by a severe, chronic, disabling condition.

A veteran of tough times I have survived paternal abuse as a child, exile that forced me to leave behind the only family that raised me and loved me, that is my uncle and aunts, the loss of my envisioned career's plans when I was stricken by Meniere's at age 22. I have also suffered the progressive loss of my hearing, and all means of sustenance after my Meniere came back after 16 years of remission rendering me disabled forever. Finally, I have lost my marriage of twenty years and yet, through it all, I have found friends who have helped me cope with all of my losses.

It is my most heartfelt desire that my story would serve as an inspiration to all patients affected by a severe, chronic, disabling condition and a celebration to all milestones conquered and their daily victories.

CHAPTER 1

— ✹ —

UNEXPECTED FALL

Alina tucked at my lab coat and nudged me gently towards the hall. I quickly took it off, washed my hands thoroughly and reached for my wallet which I stored in an old metal desk drawer. Sue and Kathy joined us. Amid laughter and a lively, quick chat we headed to the nearest elevator.

By the time we arrived at the hospital cafeteria's entrance, I felt a sudden wave of heat burning my face. I left out a quiet sigh as I tried to grab the door. Everything became blurred in front of me; I closed my eyes, lost control and *fell down* to the floor.

My unconsciousness lasted only for two or three minutes. I was rushed to the nearby examining room to be checked out by my co-workers. Kathy took my vital signs and with great relief announced that everything was normal. I stayed in the room for a few more minutes, got up and announced that I was ready to have lunch. My face was still very red but other than that I felt perfectly fine. We all ordered our meals and in half an hour we were back in our laboratory, the Tissue Typing lab, located on the eighth floor of the University of Miami (UM) Medical School in Miami, Florida.

The Tissue Typing laboratory is an invaluable part of any hospital Transplant Department. In fact, it is the place where the fate of a transplant is actually decided. It is right in that laboratory where the magic match between a donated organ and a much needed organ recipient is consciously ascertained before a second chance at life is finally granted. To be medically precise, the Tissue Typing lab blood conducts tests to measure substances on the surface of body cells called antigens. These antigens determine whether donor tissues or organs are compatible to be transplanted into another person. They are unique for each person, sort of a "fingerprint." Measuring these antigens before a transplant is performed helps to ensure as close a match as possible between donor and recipient to avoid a rejection of the transplanted organ or tissue in the future.

It was 1986. I was about to start my last semester at the University of Miami. One more course was all I needed for graduation. In anticipation of completing bachelor's degree credit requirements, I had sought employment as a part-time worker in one of the fields of my studies at UM Medical School. The Tissue Typing lab position was a great opportunity to advance in my knowledge of Immunology. My first foray into the world of job searching had guided me to the Transplant Department. I was thrilled about my new job.

The month of August is the hottest month of the year in Miami. Temperatures might reach a high of 96^0 F. Humidity makes it feel even hotter, a truly scorching heat. People try to stay indoors as much as possible to avoid profuse sweating, stickiness and dehydration. I passed out in the middle of August. Logically, I attributed it to the summer heat, the stress of a new job, a recently failed romantic relationship (actually, it was a broken engagement) and finally a possible transitional allergy to any of the chemicals and radioactive materials I used at work everyday. What else could have been wrong with a 24-year-old woman?

Soon I put the transient episode behind me and I immersed myself in my interesting work. I forgot all about my mysterious,

2

totally unexpected fall. A week passed by and I felt fine, but on the eighth day after my sudden fall, I became ill again. This time I did not lose consciousness. Instead, I was not spared from experiencing all the rage of my new spell. It seemed like the whole world collapsed in a minute. I felt a surge of heat running up my face again. I lost my balance. My living room started to spin violently around me. The lamp hanging from the ceiling in the middle of the room began a mysterious dance; I tried to focus on it. I counted one, two, three? How many lamps were there? I lost count. The lamps were emerging one after the other just to disappear in a vertiginous non-ending circle. Stumbling upon the walls, I made it to my room. I collapsed on my bed. A wave of coldness swept my whole body. My mother reached out for a thick blanket and covered me with it. I vomited for several hours in a row. Exhausted, the vertigo and vomiting eventually subsided. The macabre *swirl* was finally over.

By the next morning, I started fearing the worst. The new crisis had been too horrible to be ignored. Afraid that a very serious condition such as a brain tumor could be the culprit for my recent symptoms, I decided right then that if another attack would overcome me I would seek professional help.

August came to an end and I enrolled in my last semester at UM. I was looking forward to graduation with great excitement. I only needed three more credits to meet the required courses for my degree. For my last course before graduation I had to present a research paper on Cyclosporine-A, an immunosuppressant drug used to abort a possible transplanted organ rejection. My mentor, Dr. Laphalle Font, was one of my new superiors also. I was being trained at working both research and clinical procedures at the same time. Weekdays I worked under the direction of Dr. Font in his research lab, situated in the medical building third floor. On weekends, I worked on the eight floor doing clinical laboratory procedures for transplant recipients.

At that time, Dr. Font was pursuing the discovery of a new type of immunosuppressant drugs, called monoclonal antibodies. He taught me the process of isolating the antibodies from other chemical compounds to be tested in transplanted patients. On weekends I continued my training in the Tissue Typing laboratory performing clinical tests under Dr. Violet Aschkinks' supervision.

In late August, I re-united with my boyfriend, Jordi after a long break-up. I also had become a full-time employee at the Transplant Department during the fall semester. Being a UM full-time worker offered me the possibility to enter into Graduate School with full-tuition coverage by my employer. I wanted to pursue a PhD. in Microbiology and Immunology. The future looked brighter than ever to me and then, all of the sudden, clouds overshadowed it again.

CHAPTER 2

—— ✿ ——

FAULTY CARROUSEL

By mid-September, the strange crises increased in frequency and duration. I decided not to wait any longer. I visited a family doctor at a Hispanic clinic, very popular in Miami in 1986. Nowadays, that clinic is no longer in business. A general checkup and basic comprehensive blood tests did not raise a red flag. All my results were perfectly normal. The doctor dismissed me without major concern. It was a "transitory thing," he assured me.

The following week my brother had to carry me down the stairs of my building and rushed me to the nearest Emergency Room. I was given two shots, one for the nausea and another one for the vertigo. As soon as I stopped vomiting, I was sent back home.

Two days later I paid another visit to the clinic. This time, after reviewing all my blood tests and my vital signs, a different general practitioner pronounced the following words,

"Headaches and dizziness are the two most common symptoms in medicine".

And with that sentence, to my astonishment, he waved me away at the door. That was the end of my second medical consultation.

Dispirited, I came back a third time to the clinic. This time, I saw a very old and gentle, wise internist who assured me that my symptoms were caused either by a neurological or an inner ear condition. He referred me to the appropriate specialists and wished me good luck. The neurologist who examined me was an old, very well-mannered doctor as well. He gave me a thorough neurological checkup in his office and finally delivered his professional opinion.

"I am convinced your symptoms are not of a neurological etiology (origin). For your peace of mind I will order a CAT-scan of your head, but I assure you there is nothing wrong with your head. You need to see an ENT (ear, nose and throat specialist)."

As predicted, the head scan was normal. I had a brief moment of relief and then with horror I realized I was very ill but no doctor could provide me with a diagnosis. My illness was a mystery. I was so confused and sick that I did not know how to proceed from there on. In an era where computers where not an integral part of daily life as today; I could only turn to the traditional method of searching for an answer. I needed to direct my steps to the public library to research the mystery that had assailed me. I could not do that. I was too sick to drive anywhere. I depended on taxi cabs services to transport me to doctor's appointments. My health was worsening by the day. I resigned myself to endure the brunt of the vertigo attacks. I also made the first mistake I will later come to regret in the course of my illness; I discarded the ENT referral. How on earth could my ears provoke such horrible symptoms? That was inconceivable to me! Good Lord, how ignorant I was at that time. I paid a heavy price for my false assumption.

With an extraordinary effort on my part I finished my research paper on Cyclosporine A. I received an A on it. And that was all the excitement I was entitled to at that time. Due to my severe vertigo and vomiting, I could not attend my graduation ceremony at the University of Miami. No cap and gown for me. No graduation ring. No pictures to remember the much awaited occasion. I was deprived of hearing my name called along with my peers to be greeted by Dr. Edward T. Foote II, the interim UM president at that time. It was December 1986. I received my diploma by mail and that was that. How many more special events would I miss out in my life? Very soon, I would find the answer.

___ Mercy, what's wrong dear? Dr. Font asked me in a worried tone.

___Oh, I don't feel well. I have this horrible pressure in my ears. I can't lift my head up to tend to the column (a chromatography column I used to separate the monoclonal antibodies from the rest of the sample serum). I am losing my balance! ___ I exclaimed in a soft whisper.

___ I am very sorry Dr. Font, I am sick AGAIN! Please I need help to lie down . . . quickly!

___Don't worry Mercy. I'll call Norma upstairs to help you to the staff's lounge. I'll be right back. He said.

Norma was a new-part-time employee at the Tissue Typing lab. She was from El Salvador and had just migrated to America to escape an assassination threat promised on by certain leftist factions in her native country. I had never met her before but when she came down to the third floor to assist me; I met a wonderful, young lady who was very compassionate and understanding.

Norma wrapped her arm around my waist and very slowly we started out of the lab towards the lounge. I could not look up or down, right or left. My eyes were fixed in a semi-closed gaze to escape the much dreaded onset of vertigo and vomiting. Since I had no balance, I leaned my body against Norma's as she gently guided me out of the room.

The University Medical Building was divided into two sections. The right side of the building was the new addition to it. It was built with plenty of windows that allowed the Miami sun rays to be reflected along the new, polished, granite floors. The left side of the building was the original one. It was a dark, poorly illuminated section. For the most part, it enclosed small windowless rooms. Sometimes, the labs had small windows that face other drab buildings; a gloomy view unless you had valid reasons in your heart to fill it with joy.

All edifices together constituted the Jackson-Hospital / University of Miami conglomerate. Dr. Font's lab was located in the old building section. In fact, most of the Medical School's Microbiology/Immunology professors had their small offices and research labs located on that floor.

As I stumbled out of my lab, beads of sweat covering my face; I sensed more than seeing the presence of sympathetic teachers, researchers and their lab assistants assembled along the dark corridors. Soft, compassionate words were uttered as Norma, literally, dragged myself along the hall. Then, I heard it. As dizzy as I was, the words reached my ears very clearly,

___Poor thing.
___What's wrong with her? I heard a female voice in the distance.
___She is suffering from a Petit Mal seizure! That's what's wrong with her!

___Oh no, dear God! I pleaded myself after I heard the term. Petit mal! No, please, no epilepsy for me!

Petit Mal seizure is just one variation of several types of epilepsy. It has been substituted by the modern term of *absence seizure*. As opposed to Grand Mal epilepsy or seizures, where the patient falls down to the floor on uncontrollable convulsions, the patient afflicted by Petit Mal might appear to be staring into space with or without jerking or twitching movements of the eye muscles. Normally, Petit Mal patients do not show any emotional expressions during these attacks. These periods usually last for seconds.

-Just because I have to stare into a fixed spot in front of me with a vacant look on my face when I am seized by these attacks does not mean I suffer from Petit Mal, right?,

I reassured myself—

A few days later, Jordi's dad, a pediatrician who had graduated from University of Havana, suggested the same diagnosis. I still refuted the possibility of a neurological problem. Time will showed me that I was correct in my assumptions then.

____ "I want us to go to a special place this weekend, baby," Jordi whispered sweetly in my ears while he gently caressed my face. I want you to relax and forget about these awful past weeks. I want us to have some fun again. I am taking you to *The Forge* tomorrow. We'll have a nice dinner, we'll dance and we'll toast to your recovery and we'll forget all about your dizziness, you'll see."____

I simply nodded in agreement with delight.

As I came out of my shower wrapped in my pastel peach bathrobe, I took a glance at my outfit for the night. My black, satin blouse and evening trousers lay on top of my bed besides my golden belt, earrings and sandals. The same golden toned clutch complemented both my ensemble and my shoulder-length-honey-blonde hair. I looked at myself in my bedroom's oval mirror as I started to apply some foundation to my face.

I sighed with relief. A sense of confidence swept me all over. *I will put this nightmare behind me. Yes, I will . . . .*

The trendy, high-end, haute cuisine Hollywood—1930's era restaurant lifted up my spirits that night. The place was amazing.

I was delighted from the moment we stepped in. Jordi was in the mood to treat us to a feast that particular night. He wanted me to feel like a fairy-tale princess entranced by an unforgettable night. And he succeeded. He ordered us a bottle of Chianti 1960 Riserva to accompany his Tuscany Sirloin Steak and my Oak Grilled Filet Mignon. The famous, New York-style-dry-aged steaks were as delectable as expected. In fact, they were superb.

The Forge, located in the heart of Miami Beach was perfectly suited for its Latin up-beat music evening show. Hansen and Raul, a very popular Cuban-duo in the 80's, were the attraction of the night. After savoring our delicious Belgian Chocolate Soufflé, we stepped up to the dance floor. We swirled happily along with other young couples; dancing to the tune of both rhythmic Latin salsa and ageless, slow, romantic ballads.

I hadn't felt so well in so long. *I felt normal again, almost.* We went back to our secluded seats. We indulged in sweet talking and dreamy plans for our future together. A few moments later, I slid to the back of the restaurant to visit the ladies room. I re-applied my glossy lipstick carefully and went back to my seat. Upon my return, beside my glass, I found a beautiful white orchid, delicately wrapped in a transparent box. *My favorite flower of all.*

A note engraved in golden letters read I Love You. I felt exhilarated. Swept with love, I looked at Jordi's large, hazel-nut eyes framed by his dark hair. *Sus ojos color de menta.*

His beautiful light green eyes were the color of a genuine green-mint Cuban candy, framed by his dark beard and thick, dark eyebrows. He was the most handsome guy I had ever been with! I leaned toward him and very gently, I kissed him on his lips. The Maitre-D walked by, he smiled at us and discreetly guided his steps to the other corner of the room.

Suddenly, like a deadly tornado it completely enveloped me. I felt it coming, swift, powerful, BRUTAL; but I was hopelessly defenseless. The English Oak paneling seemed closing on me. I felt trapped, unable to utter a sound, unable to stop it. The Matisse alternating brilliant colors right across our seat joined me in a vertiginous carrousel ride. I wanted to stop it. I failed. Instead of friendly, coordinated ups and down equestrian movements I was spun into chaos. My own private carrousel lacked harmonic rhythm. I tried again. No luck, it refused to submit to any commands. It kept spinning around and around in a discordant symphony of loud, ringing noises in my ears.

I looked up to the ornate, high ceiling. The massive, expensive chandelier glowed far too intensively. Like a mischievous accomplice it joined the carrousel festivities, playing a burlesque trick on my mind. One, two, four, it kept multiplying itself with each new round. *No please, not again.* It took all of Jordi's six feet, 200 pounds and athletic, strong body to pull me out of the restaurant. I barely made it to his red Mustang. Leaning on the passenger door the retching seized me. I fought it bravely but I shamefully lost the battle. I doubled over and returned my dinner on the parking lot for what seemed an eternity.

Our special, romantic dinner ruined by an anonymous opponent, ruined by my own, faulty carrousel. Maldito carrusel. Fatigue overpowered me, and I reclined my body unto the Mustang cream-colored seats. As I closed my eyes I heard Jordi's sincere apology to the valet parking attendant and right after it,

-That was quite a scene babe. I bet those folks think that you partied too much—Jordi said very softly while gently lacing his right hand with mine.

11

-Yes, I bet they did—I felt so ashamed and so miserable I did not speak another word until I got home.

What a waste of a delicious meal!

Almost an hour passed by, I don't recollect much from there on, except that I collapsed onto my bed, begging, pleading, crying for a good night rest and no more dizziness while the tears streamed down my face burning it like fiery lava.

CHAPTER 3

❀

CLUELESS PHYSICIANS, CLEVER VETERINARIAN

The New Year began much the same way the previous one had ended: in the turmoil of uncertainty. With horror, I realized that as time has passed, my symptoms had kept escalating in their severity and length. Even worse, there was not a diagnosis in the horizon, not a *clue* to the mysterious ailment that was affecting me.

Three more weeks passed by. Although I did not have a severe crisis as the one at The Forge, I remained low-level dizzy all those weeks. I had a general malaise from dawn to dusk. I was lethargic most of the time, all my body wanted to do was remain still and do absolutely nothing. I already had started to lose interest in all the things that kept me going until that point in my life. Fear of having to live the rest of my life submitted to a capricious, totally incapacitating, elusive illness was a constant thought in my mind. I could not think clearly about anything else. Depression had started to sink its claws on me, although I did not acknowledge it at the time.

What if doctors never find a diagnosis for my condition? A name, damn it, that's all I need, a name so I get the right treatment and be done!

In a graceful attempt to bring some sunshine into my life, Jordi planned a weekend getaway trip for us. One of Jordi's uncles,

George, lived in Bartow, a picturesque, small town located in Central Florida, near Tampa. Another one of Jordi's uncles, John, had a vacation home in Bartow. On account of its stark white walls and windows and its similarity to Washington's famous presidential residence, everybody in Jordi's family called it *The White House.* That's we stayed; in a very comfortable, restful, Ante-Bellum house, tucked away from the typical commotion of our hectic, cosmopolitan Miami.

Although I did not feel up to a five hour car drive, I felt compelled to accommodate my boyfriend's request. After all, he was trying to distract me from my own misery. Mid-January was as cold as it ever gets in Florida. It was very nice weather for a car trip, a much awaited respite from Miami's typically warm temperatures. However, my enigmatic illness was lurking inside my body, ready to strike at any moment and somehow I knew it. I knew that the battle was yet far from over. What I could have never fathomed at that time was how much longer the war would last.

Bartow was a very pleasant sight to eyes in need of beauty and solace. Famous for its azaleas and grandiose oak trees, it looked very different from Miami. Most houses displayed the typical Colonial Revival architecture of early 20th century. *The White House's* massive, boxy and symmetrical structure, blended very easily in its neighborhood. It was vast and I really admired the elaborate front with its bright white multiple column porches and sunrooms.

As much as I appreciated the intrinsic historical value of my accommodations, I felt very uncomfortable my first night. I snuggled under a thick, woolen blanket at night all to no avail. I stayed awaken most of the night grinding my teeth and shivering as if possessed by a high fever. I should have sensed that my restlessness was just a bad omen for my weekend escapade.

Morning came and the sun was up shining brightly. I poured myself a cup of steaming coffee, wrapped myself in my favorite white terry robe and stepped out into the back yard. Of course my robe had to match such distinguished lodgings! Although temperatures lingered in the 40's, I felt the sun's warmth caressing my whole body and I discarded all my previous night's fears. I heard footsteps approaching, turned around and met my boyfriend with a gentle kiss on his lips. Optimistically, I headed to the guest room and got all dressed up in a very comfortable winter-white, woolen blazer to complement the matching color turtleneck sweater and my dark teal jeans. A black suede tote and ankle boots completed my outfit. I wanted to look fashionable but not too much, just enough to make a favorable impression on Jordi's relatives.

Uncle George, a retired veterinarian, and his wife Matilde were eagerly waiting to meet us. After a delicious breakfast comprised of favorite strawberry's pancakes, Canadian bacon and another cup of hot coffee we drove to Uncle's new-remodeled, recently acquired residence nearby. We were shown around the whole place, visited the goldfish pond that surrounded the periphery of the backyard, the spacious sunroom overlooking the meticulously manicured landscape, the small but cozy library and finally we were lead to the most astonishing house's new room, the orchid conservatory.

The circular shape, built on a stone base wall conservatory with its insulated glass panels and doors provided the much needed controlled climate for the thriving delicate plants. Jordi's uncle had succeeded in accomplishing a vast variety of both natural and hybrid specimens for his private collection. The greenhouse was a beautiful place to linger and I allowed myself to examine the Cymbidiums, Phalaenopsis, Cattleyas and several other species at my own slow pace. The colorful, stunning display was a feast to my eyes. Matilda regaled me with a fragrant, blooming vanilla

15

plant potted in a brown glazed clay pot and a stunning Blue Scented Sun orchid that was in full bloom as a courtesy to the cold but sunny day.

After the tour, we moved to the conservatory adjacent seating room. As I accommodated myself in the white washed wicker roomy seat, Lori, the housekeeper brought us a tray filled with mini-cuban sandwiches, mini-chocolate éclairs and our famous *pastelitos de guayaba y queso* (guava and cheese pastries). Conversation was flowing amiably. I took a bite of my pastry and a sip of the hot cocoa when I felt the ominous whirl coming at me. The white cup escaped my grip. Its impact on the terracotta-tiled floor dispersed the shattered pieces in all possible directions. My eyes were fixed. My gaze met the wall across my seat. In what seemed to an outsider a supernatural trance, I stared at the sign hung on the wall. My brain was in a fog. It engaged in a battle of its own. Two commands. *Fight the vertigo. Remember those words. Déu Pare . . . . aquesta tabla . . . tots nosaltres.*

Where have I seen those words before? I know them. I know I've seen them before. Why can't I recall, why?

"I am familiar with your symptoms. Don't get me wrong, but I've seen that vertigo in the chickens I have treated over these past years. *Meniere,* that's the correct term. *Meniere's syndrome.*"

Uncle George's raspy voice brought me back from my false trance.

"Pardon me, uncle, what did you just say?"

"Dear, you have Meniere's syndrome. It's an inner ear disease. It produces severe vertigo and nauseas. Animals get it, too. I have treated my share of chickens with that affliction. I bet my life on it. That's what's wrong with you honey."

With all due respect Uncle, do you think for a moment that I am going to believe the words of a . . . . veterinarian. For God's sake, I am not a chicken!

Out of common sense and expected, impeccable, social manners, I kept my skepticism to myself. Besides, I felt so awful, I asked Jordi to take me to *The White House* immediately without letting his family catch a glimpse of my own doubts. One more time, my ludicrous judgment betrayed me. Time would prove me the falsity of my "scientific assumptions". Time would also teach me an invaluable lesson, not to discard any medical leads without testing them first.

Meniere Syndrome. It sure was the first time I heard the word in my young life but by no means was it the last one. In fact, I heard the name again right after I returned to Miami.

CHAPTER 4

※

SORRY, NO VIP SUITE AVAILABLE FOR YOU

The phone rang. I stretched my arm out of my bed and reached for it.

"*Mi vida*, you are not going to believe this news. Hector, a co-worker of mine, has just left my desk. He came over to tell me that he's been having the exact same symptoms as you do. He went to see an otolaryngologist yesterday and the doctor told him he has Meniere's syndrome or Menier syndrome, I am not sure which way is it. Anyway, it's a very rare disease of the inner ear. The doctor's name is Osaki. Ted Osaki. His office is right there at UM. Isn't that really convenient to you? Isn't it? Oh God, this is so great. You call him tomorrow and you'll make an appointment. Hector got some pills from Dr. Osaki and he's feeling much better already. I have to go now. Bye"

And with the familiar click I stopped hearing my mom's voice.

Osaki? Is that a Japanese name? Is he oriental? How much does he/she charge per visit? I am about to exhaust all of my savings in doctors and taxi cabs fares. God, there goes my dream vacation in Brazil!

Meniere? Isn't that what Uncle George's chickens got? Did I happen to mention **that** term to my mom? Why can't I recall? Am I losing my memory, too?

I'll have to wait until Mami comes back home from work.

When my mom came back from work she told me that Hector was an old man who worked at *Vanidades*, a popular Spanish magazine editorial where my mom was a secretary in the Consumer Relations Department. Hector had been suffering from severe dizziness and loss of hearing for awhile. Dr. Osaki had diagnosed him with Meniere's disease and had provided him some pills that had brought Hector a new hope in his severely disrupted life. I immediately scheduled an appointment with Dr. Osaki for the following week totally convinced that I would finally be able to put an end to my misery. My mother also re-assured me that I had never mentioned the word Meniere to her after I came back from my trip to Bartow.

Hey, what do you know? Perhaps, chickens and I have something in common after all!

Dr. Okawi's office was located in the UM medical private offices section. It was a medical practice for insured patients or patients like I who could afford to pay $200.00 per visit, even if that meant that my scarce savings would soon all vanish. A set of auditory and balance tests were performed on both my ears and finally over the course of several weeks, and after so much anguish and sheer discomfort from all the unpleasant tests, a verdict was pronounced. I had Meniere's disease; I was officially a "Menierian".

I felt elated. It was not all in my mind after all! It was not Petit Mal. I had a medical condition that affected my hearing system. I had to get the right treatment, some pills and in a matter of days, I would be back to my daily routine and back to my plans and dreams. I left Dr. Osaki's office with some prescriptions in my hand, one for Antivert, to treat the vertigo and another one for Dyazide, a diuretic medication. A water pill was and still is standard treatment in all Meniere's patients to diminish the excess fluid volume inside the inner ear. When I got home I was shaky and distraught from the dizziness but I had a name for my illness and that was all I cared about at the moment.

"*Mi vida*, what else did the doctor tell you?"

"Ay mami, I have Meniere. It is a disease that affects the inner ear. There are some canals deep inside the ears that contain some fluid called endolymph. For those afflicted by Meniere's, this fluid increases its volume without a feasible explanation. That fluid excess provokes a rupture in the canals' membranes and the whole process causes the vertigo and nausea. In most cases, only one ear is affected. I think I fit into that category, right?"

"One ear? Okay then, which one of your ears is the affected one?"

"Well, the truth is that . . . I don't know. Dr. Osaki told me that I am an atypical case. I don't have any hearing loss. My hearing is perfect. Isn't that good news?"

"Yes, I believe so too. Did you get any pills? Yes? Oh, I see them. Okay then, I'll bring them over. Wait for me in bed. I'll be right back."

While my mom got my meds ready, I lied down in my bed and read with great interest the Meniere's literature that Dr. Osaki handed out to me earlier in the day. Prospér Meniere, a French physician, was the first one to describe the symptoms of the illness back in 1861; hence, the name of the disease. It is characterized by four typical symptoms.

-Ringing in the ears (medical term Tinnitus)

-Fullness in the ears.

-Severe vertigo episodes that might be accompanied by nausea, vomiting and loss of balance.

-Progressive hearing loss. In most patients, only one ear is affected. But in a smaller percent the disease is bilateral; it is present in both ears.

Very strange indeed. I do have all the symptoms, except . . . . loss of hearing. Can it be possible that . . . I have gotten a wrong diagnosis? Why is it so hard for me to remember some things at times?

It was very late at night and I was drained. I swallowed my meds and transported myself to dreamland. The Antivert and the Dyazide seemed to work for a while, but a month into the prescribed treatment I had to be absent from the lab for a whole week due to serious dizzy spells. Upset, I went back to Dr. Osaki's office. By then, it was obvious that Meniere's standard treatment was not meeting my expectations.

Dr. Osaki's last resource was a type of medication called scopolamine patches. The small, round patches were very similar to the Dramamine patches worn before embarking on a cruise to control motion sickness and nausea. A small, round patch was placed behind one of my ears and every 72 hours the patch was switched to the other ear. Initially, I felt some relief but my hopes were "drowned" very quickly and not precisely in the ocean waves of a luxury Caribbean cruise. After three months of the scopolamine therapy, it was obvious that the patches did not have the desired effect on me.

I came back to Dr.Osaki's office for a last time. His blunt, harsh words took me aback,
"Sorry, but I can't do anything else for you. I don't know how to control your symptoms."

Back then, I had no idea that life is like a long, long corridor full of rooms. Some are small, some are big. Some are impeccably decorated, still others are nothing but ruins and of course there are the modest-nothing fancy-full of hand-me-down furniture, nevertheless clean and neat.

Every morning, as soon as the sun rises, we start a new path down life's hall. Most of us aspire to linger in the luxury suites of life but have to be content with the more moderately priced accommodations. That is, we wake up, have a nice breakfast or a low-calorie, not-so-tasty one if we want to shed some pounds and head right away to our places of work where routine tasks await us with a relentless urgency. We meet the same people every day. We have lunch at noon and return home later in the evening just to start all over the same routine the next day. (In today's economy embracing this daily "routine" is considered a luxury, who would have thought just a few years ago?)

Once in a while there is some rewarding, exciting experience in our lives. More often than we expect, we encounter some obstacles of every possible kind. Nonetheless, we don't complain because after all, more than three quarter of people in this world live in very precarious conditions. Hey, at least we get by in the 'world's richest country" (for how long we'll we hold that title, is anybody's guess nowadays) and at the end of day, most of us plop our feet up in front of a plasma TV set with a full belly. No right to complain!

Don't mind that a small, tiny, humanly minority enjoy life at its best (at least for a while). Money, youth, good health, beauty and **love** are part of their lovely lives. Enjoy it while it lasts!

Yet, to a third group of unfortunate souls, the first two options are seldom or never available. Worn-out furniture, greasy stoves, empty, rodent-infected cupboards and bared, paint-peeling-off the walls are the typical scenario they face every new dawn. Very rarely, they can acknowledge the fact that there is a sun shining on the streets and that the sky is sometimes embellished in a beautiful array of soft, pastel colors. Very rarely, they might catch a glimpse of a sweeter life!

These people strive fiercely every morning to open up the forbidden luxury room's doors of the long gallery ahead of them. But day after day, the doors remain tightly locked; even the average rooms' doors remain elusive to them. If ajar, they soon are slammed shut furiously on their faces. Back to square one or should we say room one, the one full of misery and zero opportunities for a better life?

Slam, slam, slam!

That is the story of those who have to battle relentless, disabling symptoms in their journey through the corridor of life confronting a crushing chronic illness. That was the category I belonged to that morning at Dr.Osaki's office.

Great! I have a name for my illness. But what good is it if there is no cure or treatment available to me. Another door has closed on me. Where do I go from here?

I had no clue, but I knew I wanted a fair chance at the *Waldorf Astoria, Bora-Bora and Breckenridge luxurious lodging.* I wanted the best health I could possibly attain! I was determined to earn my own V.I.P. suite.

Norma, my friendly and altruistic co-worker offered me transportation back and forth to the lab. I appreciated it immensely. I was extremely apprehensive about driving because I never knew when I was going to be dizzy. One early morning, as I got to the hospital main entrance, I felt lightheaded. I hurried up to the entrance cafeteria and ordered myself some breakfast. The place was full to capacity as it was customary at that time of the day. I grabbed my tray and sat down to eat when the impending retching seized me. I threw up all the food on my tray to the astonishment of all the surrounding, curious customers. My pride was hurt but my head was spinning out of control. I was wheeled to Jackson Hospital ER immediately by a Samaritan soul.

As I was waiting to be triaged, I continued retching. A middle-age, skinny lady dressed in a soiled, raggedy dress approached me. She was barefoot and truly looked like a junkie, a very familiar picture at the only public hospital in Miami. I tried to evade her out of repulsion and innate fear but she handed me a basin to throw up and with a swift, totally unexpected movement from her part, she reached out for the hem of her filthy garments to cleanse and wipe out my face from my stomach's expelled contents. I felt embarrassed, not so much for her actions as for my rejection of her. I tried to stop the strange lady,

"Please don't do that," I managed to whisper

She replied,

"I don't mind at all. I am filth. I am scum. I am nobody but you; you are young, pretty, obviously a doctor or a nurse. You are dressed up like an angel in your pretty white lab coat."

A nurse grabbed my wheelchair hastily and brought me inside a private, examining room. I did not have time to say good-bye to the stranger. Stories tell us time after time that angels might appear to men disguised as common human beings. Whether this lady was as real as my doctors or an angel sent from above, this incident taught me a valuable lesson I will never forget in my life. I am no one to judge anybody else based on his outward appearance, not even by his actions. Riches, fame and social status are not a guarantee of a pure heart. Like the "good thief" this anonymous lady might enter the kingdom of heaven before many others who claim their privilege and right to do so. A precious lesson indeed.

I spent that whole day at Jackson. IV's in my veins to re-hydrate me and anti-nausea medication stabilized me again. In the evening I was released home without a valuable diagnosis. I was an intriguing puzzle to the young intern who treated me that day. It was neither the first time spent at a hospital because of my vertigo nor was it the last one either. However, after that day, I knew I had to make a painful but unavoidable decision. I had to leave my job at the lab and keep up the search to recover my health. That became my priority and obsession from there on.

CHAPTER 5

❦

UNAVOIDABLE DECISION

The following week I decided to resume work, at least on a tentatively, more flexible schedule. Norma waited for me in my building parking lot in her light green Chevy. She kissed me good morning and off we sped along the 836 Express Way congested traffic. Norma's light chat was as joyful as usual; it was a balm to me.

It was a typical suffocating summer day. As we walked from the parking lot to the Medical Building, I could smell the irritability on patients and medical staff alike passing by. It was the torrid *Miamiense* weather.

As soon as I entered the Tissue Typing Lab, I slipped on my lab coat, stashed away my purse in an old cabinet drawer and readied myself to start working. Cleaning, scrubbing, disinfecting; I was efficiently concentrated on my daily morning routine. The strong odors of the ten percent chlorine solution and alcohol swiftly began to escape through the hood extractor. One final scrub to my work bench and I went to the refrigerator in back of the lab to retrieve my patient's samples for the day. The much awaited MLC (Mixed Lymphocyte Culture) assay was arranged to begin its first steps.

MLC's are one of the utmost important tests to predict a successful outcome in a transplant. Peripheral blood lymphocytes (a type of white blood cells that produces antibodies to attack infected and cancerous cells and are also responsible for rejecting foreign tissue) from both donor and recipient are mixed together in tissue culture for several days. Lymphocytes from *incompatible* individuals, individuals who present incompatible antigens, stimulate each other to proliferate significantly whereas those from *compatible* individuals do not. That is why this assay is vital to any successful transplant.

I spent the early morning hours diligently working on my one-way MLC. Around noon, the first assay steps had been completed. It was time to inactivate the patient's lymphocytes by means of potent gamma rays emitted by cobalt radiation; thereby allowing only the untreated remaining population of cells to proliferate in response to the unique foreign histocompatibility antigens. With a firm grasp, cautiously I placed the vials containing the valuable microscopic cells in a test tube rack and headed towards the elevators. It looked like I would have a solitary ride to the basement. As the ride began, I felt the familiar sensation overwhelming me. The heat rush went all the way up from my chest up to my cheeks giving them a deceitful rosy glow. I gritted my teeth and tried to dismiss it. Tiny sweat beads covered my flushing face. I dabbed at them with the palm of my hand and fixed my eyes on the car floor. The car finally stopped. The doors jolted and I tried to regain my strength as I exited it. The corridors were deserted and the basement looked as solitary and gloomy as ever.

Jesus, this place is as spooky as it could get. No wonder basements are always featured in horror films!

I advanced to the huge radiation vault with a quick stride. I stopped in front of the thick radiation-proof doors. I gazed up above them. The Big Circle above the gigantic doors was brilliant emerald green colored. It was safe to pull the heavy doors open. I walked down to the center of the room and placed the cells on the sterile metal table facing the radiation rods containing the cobalt-60 pellets. The tubes seemed so insignificant in the vastness of the room and yet it was all so deceiving. To a significant percentage of patients those small crystal tubes represented the difference between years of productive life or a fast approaching, painful death.

I turned around and reached for the opposite wall. A quick click on the switch and count down began . . . only 10 seconds to flee the room before I became the collateral victim of the lethal gamma rays.

One, two, oh no, God, no!

It hit me. It overpowered me. The shrieking high-pitch pierced my head from ear to ear. My ears were so full they seemed ready to explode. Spin, my heart beat fast, spin, beat faster, somebody stop spinning my head please! My heart raced so fast I thought for a moment it was to rip my chest open and escaped its oppressive prison. The vertigo was too strong now to fight it on my own. Any remnants of denial were finally dispelled.

Please Lord. This place is deserted. Nobody can help me, not even if I scream at the top of my lungs. Please, let me reach the door. Give me strength.

I am trapped. The door is not going to open. Please!

An ultimate inner strength invaded me and I tugged at the door that yielded to my relentless grip. Slowly, the door finally closed behind me. My legs weakened and all I could manage was to press my back against the wall as I slid down to the floor. My long white coat could not shelter me from the cold chills sweeping my body. *What an irony! There's a sweltering weather outside and I . . . . I am as cold as a lost, solitary little girl caught up in a dark, winter blizzard!* I had one last distorted but accurate image before I succumbed to unconsciousness. I looked up at the Big Circle one more time. The bulb displayed an intense ruby red beam. A soft grin appeared on my face. I had escaped the effects of the most potent radiation ever known to man. I had escaped the overwhelming doses of gamma rays trying to mess up my DNA. I had escaped *CANCER*.

When a few minutes later, I woke up in the staff's lounge surrounded by the worrisome facial expressions of Dr. Font, Dr. Aschkinks, and Norma, I knew that I could not postpone any longer the painful but unavoidable decision. I could not allow placing my life in danger ever again. I could not risk compromising the University transplant patient's lives either. Lastly, although Dr. Font was the sweetest, most compassionate boss any employee could ask for, always willing to do my work when my mysterious illness hit me, I knew perfectly well that I could not tend to my position's duties any longer.

It was totally unfair from my part to keep my generous mentor and chief covering any longer for me in the lab. With tears rolling down my cheeks I signed my resignation the very next day. I embraced my co-workers, Alina, Kathy, Sue, Norma and my superiors, I took a last look at the plaque on the wall outside of Dr.Font's lab with my name on it, left out a sorrowful sigh and devastated had Norma drove me back to my apartment.

That evening, the whole world dropped on my shoulders. I had just lost my first, real important job of my young adult life, one that I had dreamt about it for so long. A job that I had embraced with great expectations to facilitate my transition to the next level of my career. My plans for Graduate School were shattered into a thousand pieces that night.

Dropping into a frightening stage of uncertainty, I paused to take a stock of my life. I realized that my Microbiology/ Immunology PhD. degree would have to be postponed indefinitely because of my ill health. I was assailed by an illness that could not be successfully treated. I mentally reviewed all my failures. They qualified to write my own "Series of Unfortunate Events."

Jordi and I had ceased to exist as a duo. Our final breakup was just as inevitable as my mysterious vertigo. I had canceled our carefully planned wedding several months ago. One thing led to another. I broke off our engagement. We reunited. Soon after we reunited, I began my-never-ending battle with Meniere. I had been coerced into a state of self-doubt in my affection and love towards Jordi. In time, my hesitation took a toll on us as a couple and the strenuous circumstances that surrounded us proved to be stronger than our love. We went our own separate ways. This time there would be no reconciliation.

It hurt. It hurt emotionally, mentally and physically. My vertigo sent me off into a downward spiral. I sank into intractable depression.

The box is unopened. The big, white, satiny box lying on my bed is still unopened. Not a shred of curiosity to see what her only daughter's wedding gown looks like? Mami did not go to St. Raymond church to meet the priest. Jordi's parents were there for the pre-nuptial parent-meeting with the pastor who is going to marry us. Not mami. She does not want to have anything to do with my wedding. What made me think that she would take a peek at my gown? I am such an idiot.

This bitter soliloquy had occurred a few months before my Meniere's onset.

Jordi had proposed to me six months exactly after we started dating. We were in love. Why delay joining our lives forever? Wedding preparations followed the proposal. I lacked expertise on the subject. I had been "transplanted" from economically struggling communist Cuba into the richest country of the world in 1980; the country where all your dreams were supposed to materialize.

Having been born and raised in a communist country I have to admit that back then, my naiveté regarding the economic world of an industrialized capitalist society was astounding. I was lost as to what a wedding entailed in America. Even worse, I was scared, terrified and with no female relatives or friends at that time to help me navigate the exciting but daunting task of planning a wedding. MY OWN WEDDING.

Even more stressful though was my mother's fierce opposition to my relationship with Jordi. It had been a constant struggle with my mom from day one. My mother's own relationships failures and lack of a family structure to extend her support dictated the course of her attitude towards my engagement.

Her story personifies the story of most Cuban exiles. My mom fled Cuba seeking a better life for my brother and me in this country. She left her native city, her brothers, sisters and everything familiar behind. She was never truthfully content again. Isolation and homesickness were brutal. She never recovered from the tragedy of leaving behind her beloved family; a tragedy shared by thousands and thousands of Cubans after Castro took power.

Soon after our arrival in America, her crumbling marriage came abruptly to an end. My father divorced her and married another lady in Venezuela. My mother's heart was poisoned. From that day on, she clung unto her job and her daughter, me, as her only life-lines of vital support.

Marrying me to a young man meant losing the emotional oxygen she desperately needed to breathe. She could not let go of her only daughter. Her own emotional sanity was hanging on the line by a very fragile thread. In her twisted, insecure mind, she needed me and she spared no recourse to sabotage my love in all imaginable ways in an attempt to keep me by her side. She failed to realize that instead of losing a daughter, she would gain a son. Apparently, my mother won the battle. I succumbed to her lack of support, brutal criticism, complete indifference and blunt opposition to my happiness.

Yes, my mother won the battle but ironically, in winning, she lost. She lost the war. And her loss was very costly. I called off my wedding in December 1985. Six months later, I had my first Meniere's attack. For the next three years, my mom had me all to herself but not as the young, healthy daughter she had envisioned to accompany in her solitude. Instead she got stuck with a very sick young lady who was unable to help her at all. My mom and I traveled together into the dark depths of despair that enveloped us for the next three consecutive years. I am convinced that my mother loved me dearly, but what a heavy price she had to pay for her selfishness and insecurity!

Looking retrospectively, I probably had lurking a Meniere's predisposition inside my body for a long time but the grinding emotional stress I was subjected to during my amorous relationship with Jordi was the catalyst that propelled my Meniere into full bloom. It became very clear to me from that moment on, that whatever was the nature of my mysterious malady, rejection and failure in my love life was the main trigger of my vertigo. Many years later I confirmed what I suspected at the time. At least in my case, stress is the number trigger of Meniere's attacks. In the long corridor of my own, private, individual life the VIP suite was denied to me.

CHAPTER 6

❦

THE MISSING CLUE

God certainly works behind the scenes. From the moment we are born until we meet Him face to face. We just live in such a hectic world we fail to acknowledge His Presence most of the time. Nonetheless, The Guy Up There is watching over us always, whether we realize it or not.

My ship was adrift in the middle of a stormy sea. Yet, God was still the Captain of my vessel (my life). He provided me with a new beacon in the obscurity of the tempestuous ocean to guide me ashore, even though I could not recognize His deed at that time. Another door was slammed shut in my face, yet God opened up a small window for me.

Dr. Osaki closed his office unexpectedly, and moved to another state leaving all his Miami patients in need of finding other specialists to replace his medical services. Hector, my mother's co-worker, found another ENT to treat his Meniere. This time, it was a very knowledgeable doctor in his field. He worked (and still does until present) at Miami's City Hospital.

I followed into Hector' steps and very soon I found myself in my new ENT's office, enduring still, the brutality of my relentless vertigo. My new physician was a very compassionate doctor, actually, an exceptional soul. As soon as he found out that I had been forced to abandon my career dreams due to my poor health, he volunteered to treat me Pro-Bono.

After an initial consultation that included a whole new set of hearing tests and an intriguing array of questions such as,

"Do you need to eat breakfast as soon as you wake up? And "Are you the type of person who needs to eat your three meals with no exceptions?"

He finally pronounced his astonishing diagnosis,

"Mercedes, you don't have Meniere's syndrome. YOUR HEARING IS INTACT. You are suffering from hypoglycemia instead, that's the real culprit for all of your symptoms"

"Hypoglycemia? The term caught me off guard completely. Of course, I knew what it meant. My medical background helped me out to decipher the terminology.

Hypo= Low, Glycemia = Glucose, sugar. Low blood sugar. That was the new diagnosis. But why on Earth, didn't any doctor mention it to me before? And why I was absolutely convinced that I had Meniere's syndrome and now, I am hearing a totally different diagnosis? What I can do to relieve my hypoglycemia if it's true that I do have it and really Mercy, do you believe that low blood sugar is the culprit of your horrible symptomatology? C'mon, that's hard to digest, isn't it? You are expecting a bigger fish, like a tumor or some genetic defect that nobody has ever heard of before, but low blood sugar? So, I don't have Meniere after all because I don't have any hearing loss? Gee, that sounds like the missing clue in a crime investigation!

The doc's words brought me back to reality.

"I will set you up for a consultation with my colleague. He has devoted many years of his life studying the correlation between low-blood sugar, migraines and vertigo. He will enlighten you on the subject and by the way, you can discard your scopolamine patches now. You don't need them anymore. Just a word of caution here, go slow. After five months of using the patches, your body has been accustomed to the medication. You might end up with severe withdrawal symptoms."

On my way out, I made up an appointment with the fellow colleague for the following week. I was utterly in disbelief of the new theory but I was desperate and therefore, willing to give it a try to the new "treatment". The next day it was time to switch my scopolamine patch from one ear to the other one. Instead of leaving the new patch for the stipulated 72 hours, I decided to leave it on for 48 hours, and the time after that for 24 hours. Finally, I could get rid of them completely.

Oh Lord, I did not have the faintest idea about what lay ahead of me. I spent the following weeks in the fog of a devilish nightmare. The most excruciating headaches in the history of headaches took me by surprise and rendered me crippled. I had never, ever, experienced such agonizing headaches in my whole life.

My mom would leave home for work early in the morning. So would my brother. I stayed home all by myself, sitting on my living room sofa in front of a TV set that I was not able to watch. Aside the headaches, I felt a heavy load over my eyes. I could not focus my vision on any point. I could not read either. I was deprived of my lifelong number one hobby! It was sheer agony. It was the worst penance I could suffer besides my horrendous physical pain. I would grab a small cup filled with green grapes and try to gulp them down to satisfy my hunger. I could not accomplish that simple task either. I was living a horror story.

I have always wondered what a drug-addict felt like while trying to overcome his addiction. My head pain was so unbearable that I compared my 'scopolamine-withdrawal-phase" to a drug addict's withdrawal symptoms. Although, I have never, ever touched any illegal drugs in my whole life, I had stored in my mind the description I had read on different articles about people trying to escape the iron grips of drugs; the bravery of those who had enough stamina and faith to escape from them. Those valiant souls have to suffer unimaginable torments as their bodies and minds got cleansed from their powerful addictions. In my imagination, my agonizing headaches had to resemble the symptoms of drug abusers going through detoxification.

My horrific headaches also transported me to my junior year at UM. Fall 1983. Pre-Med scholars were provided with "an invitation" to witness real autopsies, performed at one of Jackson Hospital's morgues. Undoubtedly, a grueling test for the future doctors to determine if they had "it" in them to become real doctors. The morgue was located in the basement of one of Jackson's old buildings. An innocent by-stander could have never guessed what sort "of trade" was performed inside those above-suspicion-looking concrete walls.

The pungent odor of formalin reached my nostrils. I took a step back in a futile attempt to escape the grips of the cadaver's preservative fluid.

My eyes got flooded with warm tears. Slowly, I twirled around the semi-obscure room covered in stale gray-metal tables contrasting with the stark white color of the pathologists' lab coats.

I adjusted my vision to the dim-lit spacious area as I regarded the corpses lying in their post-mortem rigid postures awaiting their turn to be sliced-up, measured, weighed, examined and finally sewn up to be positioned in their caskets.

An eleven year-old Asian boy with ligatures marks around his young, tender neck; the big and tall African-American guy who was severely burned, and as a consequence swollen-up and disfigured beyond recognition and finally the middle-age Caucasian woman with a through and through bullet hole in her face. All forensic cases I told myself.

The young, energetic pathologist put on a pair of latex gloves to begin his daily and macabre routine. A precise incision was made on the upper part of the woman's forehead and then with a forceful, single, quick maneuver of the doctor's hand, the cascade of brown hair was pulled off from front to back. The saw whirred and the skull was cracked open. The brain's gray matter was exposed. I inhaled a deep breath of formalin and stayed closer to the cadaver-dissection table. I knew the Head of the pathologists was watching us closely to spot a fainting prospective-doctor. Not me. I stood firm on my ground.

Scalping. Indian scalping macabre pictures appeared also in front of me. This is what it must have felt like to Indian-victims, first blundered with a tomahawk and then having their scalps removed in a harrowing, savagely move.

My head hurt. It hurt like the autopsy skull cracked-open three years ago, it hurt like the centuries-old Indian scalping accounts. It felt like my hair was being ripped-off, front to back and a hair tuft was paraded to a ferocious, cheering audience, thirsty for inflicting pain and misery. It hurt beyond description.

Exhausted I got into my shower. I let the warm water run over my head for a long, long time. The water flowed. I stood still. The water cascaded down my head and my face and so did my tears. I cried, I cried, I cried, endlessly. I could not grasp the meaning of the torment I was living. It was surreal.

CHAPTER 7

❧

THE GENIUS DOCTOR, VICIOUS MIGRAINES, LOW BLOOD SUGAR AND MENIERE CORRELATION

The early morning sky was swayed in smothering soft reds and purples. The invigorating ocean breeze from the bay bathed hospital outpatient building made my body shiver a little bit. I buttoned-up my blazer close to my chest. I felt cold and I was blinded by my vicious headaches. I hurried up my stride. I managed to find my way to the new doctor office. He shook my hand and I sat in a comfortable aged-leather chair right across his desk.

Although this fellow colleague doctor was born in Germany, he spoke Spanish very fluently with a very soft, rhythmic accent derived from years of living both in Spain and in South America. He also spoke English and his mother tongue very fluently but from the very first time we met, we carried-on all of our conversations in my native language, Spanish.

Dr. Genius (as I shall refer to him from now on) spent most of his early life in Spain. It was there that he earned his undergraduate degree in chemistry in 1935. He then returned to Germany to work toward his Ph.D. He also studied medicine. He completed all required courses in the field of medicine except for his final surgery exams. Although he did not receive a medical degree, he obtained his PhD in Biochemistry. This would prove to be the most suitable option for his future endeavors. Hi vast knowledge of Biochemistry enabled him to elaborate his famous research breakthrough study some years later.

In 1937 he went to South America as a professor at the National University of Colombia, where he taught physical chemistry and other subjects. In 1957 he was appointed president of a very famous university in Colombia. He acted as a Ford Foundation adviser in science and technology until 1975.

"Mi querida niña, (My dear girl, he used a very common expression used in Colombia when speaking to a young, unmarried lady) after reviewing your hearing exams and your history of vertigo I can assure you that you are a hypoglycemic person. You see, your pancreas is producing too much insulin, much more than what is supposed to. Such an overactive pancreas is triggering a set of chemical reactions in your body that end up in severe vertigo like the ones that you have been suffering for a while. It is the same pattern that you find in migraine sufferers, ah, don't you suffer from migraine headaches?"

"No, not really."

"Oh well, my study about low blood sugar levels has been performed in migraine sufferers only but it has been well established that migraine and vertigo, especially Meniere's vertigo goes hand in hand as well. I promise you that if you follow all of my instructions you will most likely be relieved of all your episodes."

I looked inquisitively into the pair of steely blue eyes gazing at me. Dr. Genius' charming personality captivated me from our first meeting. His amazing, vast and profound expertise in the field of medicine and biochemistry earned my admiration forever. In due time, it was his sweet, compassionate and genuinely, humble character that won my heart for the rest of my life. Anxious to hear about a possible cure for my enigmatic affliction, I proceeded to listened to his study regarding migraine headaches, low blood sugar and their relationship to Meniere's syndrome.

Many scientists involved in research gravitate to a particular field because their lives have been touched personally by it. That was such the case with Dr.Genius personal interest in migraine headaches. Initially, he became interested in migraine for personal reasons: he, too, was a migraine sufferer.

"You see Mi niña, when I was twelve years old I experienced my first migraine attack. Some years later my attacks intensified in frequency. Although my work as a professor gave me a great deal of satisfaction, it was considerably hindered at times by my recurrent migraine episodes. Alarmed, I consulted many different specialists and psychologists, all to no avail. Angry at myself, I decided to "grab the bull by the horns" and conduct my own research to discover the cause of my migraines. Thank God, I succeeded."

"How did you do it? I asked him.

"Well, as you know migraines are characterized by a recurrent, throbbing headache of variable duration, intensity and frequency, a headache that is often preceded by visual disturbances, aversion to sound and light, nausea and occasionally vomiting. When the actual pain begins, it is usually localized in one side of the head, but not always. In severe cases, patients have tingling sensations and lose sensibility in the lips, the tongue and sometimes the face. Memory and reasoning might be impaired for awhile. The attacks might last from hours to several days and of course, not all patients exhibit all these symptoms at the same time. I should inform you that I have been the victim of all these symptoms at different times during my whole life. But I know you are most interested in your specific condition. Am I right?"

"Well, I suppose, but when did you begin your migraine study?" I asked him.

"In 1961, I began my experimental research in the laboratory of Biochemistry at a Medical University in Bogotá partially funded by Foundation Grants. I have devoted twenty years of my life proving that migraine headaches are directly related to low blood sugar levels and in genetically predisposed people they are a consequence of an overactive pancreas. The excess insulin produced by this endocrine gland enhances the secretion of opposing hormones, catecholamines, such as adrenaline and norepinephrine which are vasoconstrictors and in turn stimulate the production of vasodilator chemicals known as prostaglandins. The latter are ultimately responsible for triggering a migraine attack."

At that point, Dr. Genius showed me a series of charts indicating high insulin production in dozens of migraine sufferers whom he had tested and advised for relief of their headaches. After looking at the charts very carefully, I asked him,

"Doctor, you are talking about a pancreas that produces too much insulin. That is the opposite of diabetes, right?"

"Yes, excess production of insulin is the opposite condition of diabetes."

"Well, if migraine headaches are the result of insulin overproduction and consequently low blood sugar, what is the treatment to cure it? And how does that affect my vertigo?"

"Well, my dear, there is no cure per se but my treatment which consists of a diet rich in natural carbohydrates, such as rice, pasta, and breads are sufficient to control the hypoglycemia. However, the diet must be absolutely devoid of refined sugar (sugar that has been obtained through chemical processes like in the case of common sugar) and meals should be taken at strict intervals of no more than three or four hours. You see, instead of having three square meals a day, the meals should be divided into smaller portions like six or seven times a day. The regimen is not difficult. Over 90 percent of migraine patients who have followed my advice have been relieved of their migraines permanently."

"Excuse me, but what exactly do you mean by a diet of devoid sugar?"

"It is very simple, besides the obvious sweets and desserts; migraine sufferers should avoid all foods that have listed sugar, molasses, honey or corn syrup as part of their ingredients. You need to be extra careful and read all labels before you purchase any foods. Don't fall into the trap of believing that because a label reads sugar-free, it is necessarily so. Sometimes, a sugar-free label may list dextrose as one of its ingredients and that is kind of confusing for most consumers.

"I will give you another example, you also have to take into consideration the artificial sugars you use in your beverages. Aspartame is fine to use but beware of "Equal". If you read closely the tiny package label, you will see that equal contains both saccharin, which does not affect the glucose levels and . . . dextrose. Therefore, here we go again, you need to exercise caution and read every label."

Note: nowadays, many years after this conversation took place we have new artificial sugars in the market. Most diet sodas are sweetened with SPLENDA. TRUVIA AND STEVIA are also new products. Truvia is extracted from the stevia plant. Since

Dr. Genius, unfortunately, has long passed away there is no reals scientific data to document the exact effect these new sweeteners exert in migraine patients. As for me, Splenda DOES NOT induce a migraine attack when I consume products sweetened with it.

"Well, I know what you mean; dextrose is another chemical name for glucose. If a food label lists dextrose as one of its ingredients it just means that it contains glucose. That food has sugar in it! Dextrose is called that way because its solution deviates polarized light to the right; a behavior that helps to differentiate it from other types of sugars. I remember this concept very well from my Biochemistry class at Havana University Medical School before I came to live in this country."

"Exactly, you have the correct idea. For example, mayonnaise, catsup, cereals and most salad dressings contain refined sugar. I should also mention that alcoholic beverages must also be avoided, especially the most concentrated ones. Sweet wines and liqueurs almost always precipitate an attack, because they contain two hypoglycemic substances, sugar and alcohol. They are a lethal combination. Beer is by far the most detrimental alcoholic beverage to a migraine patient. It contains maltose (a type of sugar), alcohol and oxalic acid. They all have the ability to stimulate the pancreas to produce excess insulin and therefore lower the blood sugar levels. Stay away from it!"

"Doc, this is really a very interesting theory but I still want to know how low blood sugar affects me directly."

"It is estimated that about 28 million Americans have classic migraine headaches. In a room with a hundred people, thirteen are likely to have this ailment. Now, there are other studies that show that presence of migraine in patients with Meniere disease might be up to 56 percent. In patients with bilateral Meniere, where both ears are affected by the disease, the prevalence of migraine might be up to 86 percent. As you can see my dear, there is a strong correlation between both diseases. Therefore, it is safe to assume that low blood glucose levels or hyperinsulinemia (overproduction of insulin) might have an important role on the onset of Meniere vertigo."

"I understand, but your colleague told me I do not have Meniere's disease because I have not lost any hearing so far!"

"You are correct, but since you have all the other typical symptoms of a Meniere patient, I strongly suggest that you follow all my instructions regarding my hypoglycemic diet and then we shall meet again in two weeks to discuss your progress."

I left Dr. Genius' office with a new found optimism and the resolution to start the new regimen as soon as possible. The following two weeks I experimented with new foods and I tried to follow all the dietary instructions as indicated. Thankfully, my tormenting headaches started to vanish but my dizziness continued in spite of my best efforts. The following meeting with Dr. Genius took place in a more relaxed and un-conventional setting. We discussed "my progress" or lack of it, over lunch at the hospital's cafeteria. Over a typical American lunch that consisted of a hamburger, French fries and a *diet soda*, I told Dr. Genius that my dizziness continued in the same pattern as before. Dr. Genius instructed me to avoid medications that might contribute to lower blood sugar levels. He also handed me out a copy of his recently published book. He advised me to read it very carefully and to adhere to all the rules stated very explicitly in it.

Three more weeks passed by and I still found myself in the same predicament as before. I arranged a third meeting with Dr. Genius. Although I acknowledged that I have been very fortunate to meet personally a true genius in the medical field, I had to admit to myself that Professor Genius discovery had failed to provide a cure for my vertigo. His diet was of no avail.

At our third meeting I received some news that took me completely by surprise. Dr. Genius confided in me that in very few cases the real culprit of an overactive pancreas was a tumor called insulinoma. Although, its occurrence was very rare and it was seldom malignant, it could be fatal if not removed promptly. To my dismay, I also found out that no MRI or CAT scans could detect insulinomas. I had to submit myself to a rigorous, closely monitored fasting for 72 hours to rule out the possible presence of an insulinoma in my pancreas. Every two hours a vein blood a sample would be obtained and analyzed for glucose, insulin and c-peptide levels. At the end of the test, very low glucose levels and high insulin levels would confirm the presence of the tumor. To make matters even worse, Dr. Genius recommended me to be very selective regarding the endocrinologist I would consult for such an uncommon test. A knowledgeable doctor in this particular field was of utmost importance to the success of the experiment.

I had the formidable task of looking for a reputable physician who would be willing to administer me the insulinoma test. Alarmed by the recent news, I headed straight home.

A tumor, just what I need in my life. A tumor at my age. Fasting . . . for 72 hours?

I would never survive this test. Oh God, how am I going to do this? How can it be that I have a tumor in my pancreas? What if I die? I am terrified.

CHAPTER 8

❦

THE UNTHINKABLE

In the medical field, it is fashionable to place a great deal of emphasis in a possible psychological origin for illnesses that are particularly difficult to diagnose. These conditions are often referred as *psychosomatic disorders.* Scientists believe that deeply rooted, unresolved traumas might manifest themselves through different well-established physiological symptoms. Although the aforementioned theory is valid in some patients, i.e. Post Traumatic Stress Disorder (PTSD), it was very difficult for me to believe that my real symptoms could be "in my mind" as some well-intentioned friends suggested to my mother.

A few months before I met Dr. Genius, I decided to accommodate my mother's desire to consult a psychologist at the Miami Psychology Institute. My case was assigned to a therapist by the name of Judith Lear. Judith was tall, slender and in her mid-thirties. She had long, black hair and a wide, affable smile. We never got deep into her personal life, but I soon learned that she was a divorced mother with two young children.

Our first session lasted an hour and a half. Although I answered all her questions as truthfully as possible, we only discussed the most general and obvious facts of my life. At our second meeting I started recounting some of my most painful memories and fears. I told Judith about my broken engagement, the inevitable ending of my most significant love relationship in my young life and my mother's fierce opposition to my relationship with Jordi which downplayed a pivotal role in our final separation.

I told her about the long awaited graduation ceremony I missed when I received my bachelor's degree, my ongoing battle against the uncertainty of my incapacitating vertigo and yes, about my harrowing journey through the Florida Straits in 1980 when I left Cuba via the Mariel Flotilla. I told her about how my overloaded yacht with refugees began to sink in the middle of a frightening sea storm just 30 miles away from my country. I recounted the story of how a USA Navy aircraft carrier vessel rescued me and when my seasickness finally subsided; I was taken to the ship's deck and boarded a helicopter that transported me to Key West. Finally, I told her about the void in my heart and my homesickness, about how much I missed the love of my uncle and my aunts who had raised me in Cuba and whom I was absolutely positive I would never see again in my life as a result of the regime's severe migration policies.

During my third visit, Judith asked me,

"Mercedes, is there anything else from your past, possibly a history of abuse that you have not mentioned to me yet?"

"Yes, there is, in fact . . . . there I trailed off and finally, I said resolutely,
Yes, my father abused me from the time I was eight years old until I was twelve but I do not want to discuss this issue any further."

Judith respected my wish but from that day on, every single time we'd meet, she would tell me,

"You are carrying a massive emotional and psychological baggage with you wherever you go; a heavy load in your heart. It is about time to lighten it up."

Unfortunately, Judith never explained how I was supposed to extricate myself from my heavy emotional baggage. Perhaps it was the way psychology is supposed to help patients to work through their own emotional traumas, but I was lost in the middle of nowhere and there were no signs of which route I needed to travel. I did not have a road map traced out for me, nor what kind of articles to carry in my luggage to accompany me through my life journey. I was completely disoriented. After a year of weekly consults with Judith, I knew I was not remotely close to an answer. My distressful symptoms were present as ever. I decided to explore other avenues.

Even though I felt like a cartoon character standing in front of a sign, scratching her head, while gazing at a sign with the name of a town written on it and many arrows all pointing in different directions, I had to keep on my search for an answer. I needed to find an endocrinologist to decipher the "insulinoma enigma."

The *chosen one* was a specialist whose office was located in Hollywood city, near Miami. With an incredible effort on my part; I drove down to Hollywood for about an hour to meet Dr. Paul Jenkins one early June morning. He heard my story and ordered a fasting glucose test to see where we were standing regarding my glucose levels. When Dr. Jenkins reviewed the results of the glucose test, he metamorphosed himself into a modern version of Dr.Jekyll/ Mr.Hyde.

Although he recognized that my glucose results were on the lowest side according to the parameters set out to measure normal blood glucose levels, he dismissed me as a hypoglycemic patient altogether. According to him, the sugar levels were not low enough to warrant an insulinoma test. In a verbal tirade, that I will never forget, he blamed all of my symptoms on the typical

"It's just your nerves. Why are you hyperventilating now? What happened to you in the past that you are hiding it from me? Why are you such a nervous wreck? You just need to see a psychiatrist; there is no need to waste any more of my time. And to my astonishment, I was ushered out the door before I could reply to any of Dr. Jenkins's questions. (Or should I call him Dr. Jekyll?)

"Jerk, jackass, you made me drive all the way down to your office for nothing, just to blame my vertigo on my nerves?" You have a lot of nerve, idiot!"

Back in my apartment I knew my quest for an answer was far from over. The following days found me dizzy as hell. In spite of my misery, I managed to talk over the phone to Dr. Genius. He helped me to compose a very detailed letter explaining all of my symptoms to send to selected specialists to evaluate if I was a good candidate for a 72 hrs. glucose test.

I scanned some endocrinologists' names in a medicine textbook used by UM Medical students. I decided to send a missive to an ENT who lived in California and to another one with an office established at Emory Hospital in Atlanta. I sent out a third letter to the Office of the US Surgeon General in Maryland.

Nowadays, it would have been a piece of cake to look up those names in the web and contact the doctors by electronic mail. Back in those days, I had to settle for the customary "snail mail" and wait patiently for an encouraging reply. Do you know that popular saying from Atlanta? That in order to sing the blues you need to be suffering? Well, let's just say that if I would have been a blues singer I would have received a standing ovation for my singing.

Meniere was in full swing. I endured nausea, retching, vomiting, imbalance, the whole room spiraling out of control. Round and it round it went, over and over. I had to crawl on all fours to make it to the bathroom and hugged the toilet for what it seemed years. I succumbed to utter despair.

Unexpectedly, depression seized me like never before. It sent me down to a black hole where there was no hope, no solution, and no more strength to keep on searching for a meaningful life. Almost three years of agonizing suffering, countless doctor's visits, exams and treatments finally took a horrendous toll on my nerves.

And then, the unthinkable happened. I attempted to end my young, meaningless life, not once, not twice but *almost* three times. People say that you commit suicide. I beg to differ. You commit a crime; you are a victim of suicide. My head was inundated by shrieking and screaming demons; my own made-up demons. *There is no use. Nobody knows for certain what's wrong with me. I am lonely, my relatives have turned against me; all of my friends have abandoned me. I lost my job; I lost the love of my life. I am suffering unbearably. You got nothing going on for you girl, NOTHING!*

I knew I had to stop them; I knew they were absolutely right. My life had no purpose whatsoever. It was not worth it to continue with it.

It is not my personal intention to dwell into the specifics of my desperate behavior at that time of my life. I just want to emphasize that in spite of my best efforts, I failed to give patience and hope another chance

God, I am so cursed that I am deemed to suffer endlessly. I am not even capable of . . . All my medical background and I can not even help myself? Pathetic! What a loser!

I waited and waited in bed until I heard the door slammed shut. My brother had just grabbed his electrician tools and left for the day. My mom had preceded him already. I went to my bathroom and I retrieved a shaving razor from the medicine cabinet. Standing in the middle of my small bedroom, I grabbed the razor with my right hand and brought it near my left wrist. I vacillated. I did the same maneuver again. I paused. As I lifted up the razor for a third time, something unexplainable occurred. Whether it was my innate desire to continue living, a desperate cry for another opportunity at life or an invisible force, I violently threw the razor on my bed and kneeled down by it. I brought my hands together in a supplicating prayerful gesture and I let the words hidden in my heart escape from my lips. I needed help, desperately and there was only one person who came to my mind to hear my plea.

Lord, I know you are The Only One who can help me. Please forgive me for attempting to end the life that you gave me but I don't know what else to do. I know you are Omnipotent and nothing is impossible for You. Just like you healed the crippled man by the Bethesda pool, I beg You to heal me too. Lord, You are alive. You are powerful. You are merciful; take compassion of me and restore me back to health. I acknowledge that no one, absolutely no one in this world loves me the way You do.

Please Jesus, You are my last resource.

Help me!!

And as soon as I verbalized all the anguish and pain buried inside my heart, I heard a startling noise. The door was thrown open and my brother and a friend came into the apartment. I dried up my tears the best I could and scurried under my comforter to pretend I was asleep. I don't recall where I hid the razor; but I remember very clearly my thoughts at that specific time. *My plans have been thwarted. They would have to be postponed; indefinitely.*

God's mighty hand prevented me from closing the book on my life when there were still many blank pages to be filled. It took me a long time before I could finally grasp that His Divine plan for me had just begun to unfold.

CHAPTER 9

❀

MEETING A SAINT

Seventy-two hours later, the bright red kitchen phone rang. My mother answered it and handed the receiver to me.

"It's my friend Blanca. She works at the office with me. She wants to talk to you about an invitation to the beach and a healing Mass. Please talk to her."

"A healing Mass? What in the world do you mean by that?"

"I don't know either. Please talk to her."

Blanca's high-pitched voice greeted me on the other end of the receiver

"How are you, Mercy? Listen, your mom has told me all about your endless struggle with vertigo. She is very concerned about you and I really would like to help."

To my amazement, Blanca questioned me about certain issues which struck me as a kind of odd interrogation.

"Mercy, do you like the beach?"
"Yes, I do."
Are you Catholic?"
"Yes, I am."

"I understand you have been homebound for quite a lot time, haven't you? How would you like to go with me and some friends to a healing Mass next Sunday at Pompano Beach and from there head on to Hollywood Beach?"

Now, wait a second, I have not been to Mass in a long time, but I used to go quite frequently when I was a child and I have never heard of such a thing as "a healing mass." What is it exactly?

"Oh, don't worry about it. You'll love it! There would be a very nice music and the priest will pray especially for all the present sick people."

"Okay then. Pompano Beach is far away from my house. I am very dizzy daily. I am pretty sure I won't make it to church, much less to the beach. I have not been able to swim in almost three years! I replied.

"That's exactly why you need to go dear. You've been way too long confined in your house, lying down on your bed, watching the ceiling whirling around and around forever. It's time for a change of scenery."

"But . . . . but I can't, you won't be able to help me."

"Yes, we will. By the power of the Holy Spirit, I promise you that my friend and I will get you to Mass and after that we will help you to the water. We'll pick you up next Sunday at 9:00 a.m. Be ready!"

Click. My breath escaped slowly. I had not felt such joy in a long time. The vast sea, colorful flowers and healthy, cute babies had always been the three most astonishing examples of God's perfect creation in my mind. Having been raised in Cuba I had been surrounded by pristine, sandy beaches for seventeen years. My high school was located right across a small beach in northern Havana. During summer time, my friends and I went to school wearing our bathing suits under our uniforms. We would wait for the bell, cross the street, strip off the school clothes and swim freely in the clear, azure waters of our little paradise.

The possibility of having some normality in my life and being able to enjoy my favorite sport again was a powerful incentive to accept Blanca's invitation. I am not so proud to admit that the spiritual aspect of our upcoming meeting did not have the same weight on my decision.

The church was full to capacity. I had never been to a Mass before where there were actually no seats available. I just had to be content to watch the Mass from a huge screen in the back of the building. It was the only way I could see the priest's face. Mass started at 11:00 a.m. sharp. It ended two and half hours later. The first half-hour of the liturgy was filled with beautiful, loud songs and praises. I had no idea that music like that could be sung in church. It really blew me away! Everybody clapped, sang and praised the Lord. The whole scenario was absolutely new to me.

The priest was preaching his homily. I wasn't focused at all. I was just going through the motions. Suddenly, I heard the words, "and the Lord says to you today, *You who are weary, you who are burdened, I tell you now, I am giving you a new life today. You'll meet new people, new friends who will have a great impact on your life. Trust in me with all your heart"*.

I left the church exhausted and starving. I felt extremely weak but a small, tiny seed had been planted in my heart. My old friends had deserted me. I had been isolated from the rest of the world for the past three years. The priest's prophetic words gave me a new

57

sense of joy and hope I had not felt in a very long time. Blanca became a solid beacon in my life from that day on. The Lord kept his promise.

Hollywood Beach was simply delightful. Blanca and Ines her friend, helped me out to the water as they had planned it. It was exhilarating to feel the refreshing water on my body again. No swimming though. I just let the waves bathe me with their rhythmic undulating movement. It felt like a piece of heaven had been sent down to me from above. Somehow, I made it back home. It was the end of August 1989.

Three days later, Blanca and Ines invited me to a prayer group named Christ the King. The group met every Wednesday at a location near my house. Carlos and Sarah were the leaders of the group. They belonged to the Charismatic Renewal Movement, a very popular movement that had been very active within the Catholic Church since 1967. Each single week, the group opened its doors to allow its members and newcomers to sing praises to the Lord and to study His Sacred Word, the Bible. From day one, I was attracted to the joyous praises and singing expressed very spontaneously at each meeting. Every Saturday, the group met at Our Lady of the Divine Providence Catholic Church for the official weekly mass.

On Saturday, September 2nd, 1989 I went to mass for the first time with my new prayer group. At the end of the service, Blanca told me,

"Mercy come here, I want to introduce you to a *Chinese friend* of mine."

I greeted a minuscule Asian-looking-Spanish-speaking-guy with a broad smile. I extended him my hand as he said,

Mucho gusto, (nice to meet you) my name is . . . . Well, all I could think of was, *dear God, how short is this man!* Little I did know at the time that that short man would be my future husband and the father of my children.

From then on, every Saturday I would slip into the same routine. I would wait anxiously all day long until evening. By then, Blanca would pick me up, we would go to Mass and after it was over we'll pay a visit to a nearby, trendy Cuban restaurant for some friendly chatting and much awaited refreshments. I totally looked forward to my Wednesdays and Saturdays outings. They were my only opportunity to be in contact with other human beings besides my mother and my brother. God was providing me with a welcomed respite from years of seclusion.

Wednesday, the third week of September 1989, I went to the prayer group as usual. Nausea, dizziness and the loud shrieking noise in my ears were rampant on that particular day. As soon as I stepped in, I wanted to go back home. Suddenly, Blanca approached me,

"Mercy on the 29th, the first Charismatic Conference in Tampa will take place. Almost everybody in the group is attending.

Fr. Tardif will be celebrating healing services for the sick throughout the whole weekend. You can't miss it!"

"Are you out of your mind?

Tampa is far away from Miami. A five-hour road trip is too risky for me in my present condition. I feel drained, unstable, dizzy and nauseous. I can't travel that far! Besides, my savings are depleted. Doctors and taxi's fares have left my pockets empty. I can't afford the bus ticket or the hotel accommodations!"

"Don't fret Mercy. I'll take care of everything." Blanca did not even bother to request my mother's help. Her attitude was resolute. Her spirit was a true projection of her generosity.

"Fr. Tardif has been endowed by the Holy Spirit with the great gift of healing. He has traveled around the world for quite awhile announcing that *Jesus is alive* and performing hundreds of miraculous healings. You can't afford not to be there Mercy!" I was far too tired of intangible medical treatments. I had no choice but to put my life in God's hands.

The hustling and bustling of people coming in and about with their traveling bags on one hand and a *cortadito* (a Cuban popular drink, half coffee/ half milk plus abundant sugar) on the other one were intolerable as was the roar of the bus' engine. I hurried into the bus and went to occupy my assigned place. It was the last seat! The small bathroom was right next to me and there was hardly any space left for my long legs. I looked for Sarah and begged her to switch my spot with somebody else's. I was the tallest lady on the bus, I was very sick; my narrow seat was an additional burden to my fragile health. Sarah wouldn't budge.

Oh, the hell with . . . . I need to make it to Tampa. I have to.

The chartered bus started to move. Pretty soon we left the city and sped along the I-75 Interstate highway. The trip was a well organized religious pilgrimage. A structured day of prayers and devotions were scheduled for its duration.

The Liturgy of the Hours, The Divine Mercy Chaplet and the Stations of the Cross were among the first to be recited. After a brief break, Sarah announced the upcoming recitation of the Rosary. I remembered my Aunt Mary kneeling down by her ample bed every afternoon at 4:00 p.m. to recite the rosary. I could not understand why she never introduced me into the practice. It just struck me then that being Catholic did not necessarily mean that you automatically are entitled to know how to pray the rosary. Certainly, not when you are a Catholic raised in a communist country.

Out of sheer compassion for my bent and twisted legs, Blanca agreed to switch her seat with me at some intervals during our trip. I found myself sitting right behind Ines. She turned around and handed me a brown wooden circle of beads with a crucifix attached to it.

"How do I use it?" I inquired.

Very patiently, Ines guided me. I was astonished. My very own first time I learned how to use an article I had seen scattered around my house in Cuba all my life. I was thrilled!

It was well into the night when we finally arrived at the local public high school where the Conference was held. I enjoyed the heart-felt praises but I felt too worn out for anything else. All I cared about was to hear the magic words "and now the Lord is healing a young woman who is suffering from severe vertigo and nausea" but the words never reached my ears.

"Oh well, tomorrow will be another day. A new opportunity to be a lucky winner in this healing lottery."

Honestly, that was all the retreat meant to me, an opportunity to win "God's lottery." I just expected to be myself a recipient of His miraculous healings. I did not have the capacity then to understand God's ways; that God treats each person exactly the way they are, like His unique creation. The mold is different for everybody. There are not hard and fast rules when it comes to God's acts. In my case, I needed more than physical healing; other areas in my life needed God's supernatural touch as well. I learned after that retreat not to put off any limits to God's favor. He is the master; He knows his business!

Saturday September 30th, 1989 was a restless night. I woke up at 5:00 a.m. just to hear Ines prank call my future husband, posing as the hotel wake-up service.

Wake-up, wake-up, wake-up, Ines repeated incessantly.

My future hubby fell for it. Not even Ines' heavy Hispanic accent was able to arouse a bit of our friend's suspicion.

"God, I can't believe how gullible this guy is."

Ines and Blanca had a good hearty laugh. I joined them. In spite of my ill health, I felt a very special bond with my new friends. We all headed to a nearby Denny's restaurant and had a delicious breakfast. I gulped down two Dramamine pills, the only anti-vertigo medication I was taking at that time. Then, we hurried up to the buses that would transport us to the retreat site.

The morning schedule was filled with songs, praises and talks. In the meantime, both corridors flanking the spacious room were occupied with long rows of laypeople awaiting their turn to reconcile themselves with God through the sacrament of Penance.

I ignored the long queues. My presence in Tampa was to regain my health back. As far as I was concerned, the Church Sacraments were not included in my agenda. Right after lunch, Blanca and I were strolling around the school surroundings. Abruptly, we encountered an average-sized old man dressed on a white-collar shirt portraying a very pleasant smile and the innocence of a child's soul in his serene blue eyes.

"Padre, qué sorpresa! Cómo está usted? (Father, what a surprise, how are you?). Blanca asked.

"I am very well, thank you, a little bit tired but in good spirits. Replied Father in his perfectly good Spanish garnished with his native Canadian accent.

"Ah Father, when are we going to have the honor of your presence in Venezuela again?"

Oh, very, very soon. Are you from Venezuela?

"Yes I am Father and I want you to know that you are very much loved and respected in my country. We can barely wait to have you at another retreat with us." Said Blanca enthusiastically.

"Oh, thank you. Thank you for your kind words."

And with a firm handshake, Father was escorted back into the auditorium. Little did I know at the time that I just had the privilege of meeting a real contemporary saint, Father Emiliano Tardif.

Saturday evening. The lights were dim. Silence enveloped the whole room. Out of deep-rooted respect, nobody dared to utter a word. The solemn procession began. Fr. Tardif donned a silky humeral veil over his white-satiny chasuble (priestly vestment) as he carried the golden-solar monstrance topped by a cross which contained the Sacred Host. His hands were covered with the ends of the veil so they would not touch the monstrance; a symbol that Jesus was really present in the Eucharist and that it was He and not his minister the one to bless and heal His people.

We kneeled and bowed our heads. The chorus led us in singing the Tantum Ergo. An occasional cough or a baby's cry were the only interruptions heard in the auditorium. The chanting ended. The Blessed Sacrament rested reverentially on the holy altar. Father took the microphone in his hands. All eyes were fixed on him.

"On this Saturday evening, day of Our Mother, let us all pray to the Virgin of Guadalupe to intercede before her son to heal all the sick people who have traveled from near and far to receive the blessings of Our Lord Jesus Christ. Tonight we want to pray for all the intentions placed in this humble basket at the feet of Our Lord. Just as the Scriptures mention that in Capernaum, the whole town came crowding Jesus and He cured many who were sick with diseases of one kind or another, we just want to present all the sick brothers and sisters gathered here tonight to Jesus himself.

Lord Almighty, look upon your children with merciful eyes, hear their plea, so tonight they receive all the graces you want to bestow on them and in return they can give testimony of your power and compassion and truly glorify your name. We also want to intercede for your children who according to Your Divine Plan are not going to be healed today. Give them an extra portion of your strength so they do not dismay in their faith and remain close to You in their sufferings. By the power of your Passion and Resurrection, heal all sadness, painful memories, traumas from the past and piercing resentments and fears settled for years in your children's hearts. Free your people from the slavery of all vices, deadly addictions . . . ."

My silent mind freed from the onslaught of all worldly thoughts dissolved into a blessed, blacked-out oblivion. Inadvertently, a salty stream started flowing out of my eyes, intensively, copiously, uncontrollably. I had cried endlessly in the past; fears, anguish, physical, emotional pain; they all had caused desperate crying spells formerly. However, this emanation of my soul was anew.

With each outpouring my heart was being renewed, cleansed and lightened.

"And the Lord keeps healing His people. There is a young man here tonight who suffers from epilepsy. Your body is very warm right now. In a few weeks you shall visit your doctor and confirm that you have been totally cured from your seizures. Then, you will give your testimony in your prayer group for the glory of God . . ."

Somebody passed me a white handkerchief to no avail. It kept coming in calmed abundant waves. How long did I cry? I've never known with certainty. Eventually though, the moist curtain occluding my eyes began to diminish, the purging was finalized and the flood gates were tightly shut. The catharsis was complete.

Not a word, not a visual image, just me and this gently, loving inner peace embracing me and kissing me. Stillness, quiet, happiness.

For the first time in my life, I cried tears of Joy!

Sunday was the last day of the retreat. Confessionals were improvised along the corridors. Folding wooden-chairs had been pulled together in pairs trying to provide some kind of privacy for the busy clericals assisting Fr. Tardif to minister the Sacrament of Reconciliation to the penitents filling out to capacity the auditorium halls. I waited patiently in line for my turn to reconcile myself with God. How long did I stay in that line?

I don't know, perhaps one or two hours. In any case, the time seemed very short compared to all the years that I had been separated from my church. Fifteen years! That morning though, God was inviting me with open arms to close the gap for all those years that we had been kept apart. Silently, I rehearsed a very detailed list of all my sins accumulated during the span of those long fifteen years.

Ave María Purísima. When was the last time you have been to confession my daughter?

Fifteen years Father.

Father, the first sin I want to confess is that when I was 13-years-old I stopped believing in God altogether.

My daughter, if that were the case you would not be sitting here in front of me this morning begging to be reconciled with Our Lord. *You never stopped believing in God!*

The rest of the day dissolved very quickly in the anticipation of the Retreat Closing Mass. Standing in the Communion queue, my mind wandered off freely. I closed my eyes and I was seven-years old all over again. I saw them vividly in front me. A blur of white clothing was sweeping in front of my eyes. The huge mahogany armoire doors were dimly illuminated in the semi obscurity of my parish, St.Augustine. Daylight was fading quickly and the few bulbs sparingly located on the church's basement ceiling were not enough to provide a clear view.

The familiar scent of anti-moth sachets invaded my nostrils. I heard the clanging of the wooden hangers as I hurriedly slipped my small hand through them separating the boys' suits from the girls' dresses.

"Hurry up honey!" My Aunt Mary called out pressuring me into making my selection. I took a quick glance and grabbed a white organza tea-length dress with short sleeves and a flowing skirt sewn in crinoline for fullness, a pair of short lace gloves and a two-tiered veiled satin tiara. Needless to say, that all those outfits belonged to the bygone era of a Pre-Castro society where freedom of religion was an undeniable right of every Cuban citizen.

The flashback intensified. I felt the cold granite pressing against my crossed legs while sprawled on the living room floor. My brother was sitting next to me, a mirror image of my pose. I saw Irma, my young, tall, teacher with her flawless creamy complexion and her long, flowing blonde hair. Every week she discreetly came to our house and instructed us in the basics of our Catholic faith to prepare us accordingly for the day when we would receive the Eucharist's Sacrament for the first time.

It was the year 1967. I was only six-years-old and my brother was eight. Even at our tender age we had deciphered on our own that our Catholic upbringing separated us from the rest of our classmates and friends. No other families in the neighborhood had their children in CCD classes anymore for fear of repression and scorn by Castro's government agents. Cubans in their vast majority had renounced the practice of traditional religion, at least out in the open. However, in spite of the brutal religious repression through various direct means such as forced exile, labor concentration camps such as the UMAP, and in many cases long time imprisonment or more subtle but effective repression methods such as denial to universities or careers with social impact, there were still brave souls like Irma willing to risk it all for the kingdom of God. There were many brave souls willing to risk it all to spread Jesus' way of live, a life of love. Many of those souls had been forced into a double life of secrecy like the first Christians meeting in the Catacombs, Irma was one of them.

My mind switched to a more pleasurable script. I remembered the beautiful, marble staircases that conducted me to the church entrance. I looked at myself in awe. All I could see was my First

Communion dress. And I in it. Receiving the Body of Christ for the first time.

The Body of Christ, said Fr. Tardif

Amen, I replied.

Welcome back my daughter, welcome back. I have been waiting for you earnestly.

Thank you, Lord. Thank you for your unconditional love. I love you, too. I whispered in the secrecy of my heart to Jesus.

I arrived home the next day, Monday at 4:00 am. I was exhausted and crashed on my bed. My new friends only had two hours left before leaving their home for work. I resented not being able to hold a job like them. Instead, I was bestowed with the "return of my previous savage headaches."

I spent the next few days dazed, bleary eyed and throwing up every few hours. I had plenty of time on my hands to reflect on my weekend—the retreat experience. No, my most ardent wish had not been granted. My headaches and dizziness were a remainder that my disease was still thriving inside my body. Nonetheless, I had had the privilege to meet one of the most extraordinary Catholic priests of all times. On the bus ride back, Eprah gave me some literature about Fr. Tardif. I read it avidly with an extraordinary effort on my part.

Fr. Tardif was born in Quebec, Canada in 1928. He joined the Missionaries of the Sacred Heart at the tender age of 21and was ordained a priest in 1955. In 1956, he left Quebec to be a missionary in the Dominican Republic. In 1973, after years of indefatigable work and very little rest, he fell sick with pulmonary tuberculosis. He had to go to Canada to be urgently hospitalized. The prognosis was dire. His disease was so advanced that there was no cure; perhaps after a year of intense medical treatments he could be discharged to await death at home.

Father recalls at that time, "After several tests were taken on me, even before the physicians started given me any treatment, I received a visit of five lay people from a charismatic prayer group in Quebec. At first, I was embarrassed to have some lay people prayed for me. I had mocked and ridiculed the charismatics for so long back in the Dominican Republic! However, out of common courtesy and respect I allowed them to lay their hands and pray for me in my hospital room and the Lord healed me thoroughly within three or four days. I left the hospital in perfect health, which I still enjoy many years later!"

After his healing, Fr. Tardif started to study the Catholic Charismatic Movement and to take part in retreats and conferences to spread the New Pentecost the Lord had bestowed in His church. In 1973, the Lord gave Father Tardif the charisms of healing and knowledge to accompany his evangelization work. In 1974, he went back to Dominican Republic, which lead him to preaching retreats on the five continents; his message is the one Jesus commanded him to share, that "Jesus is alive and still today accomplishes miracles and wonders just the way He did 2000 years ago."

Father Emiliano Tardif was one of the greatest healers of all times; his masses were extraordinarily overcrowded. Hundreds of healings have been attributed to him, many of which have been carefully documented. Among those healings are many cases of those people with terminal cancer and AIDS.

In 1980 Father Tardif founded a new community, Servants of Living Christ. The mother house is in Santo Domingo but the community has spread to other countries as well. He is also the author of books such as *Jesus is Alive* and *Jesus is the Messiah.*

Fr. Tardif's witty, down-to-earth sense of humor was a very attractive charisma that also drew enthusiastic *crowds* to his masses and retreats. It was impossible to witness his innocent, extremely funny, yet full of God's powerful preaching without having a hearty laugh. Nevertheless, as impressive as his healing and social grace were, the character quality that impacted my heart the most about his persona was his genuine, transparent humility. It did not matter how 'miraculous' a cure was obtained through Father's intercession. He remained the same, simple, modest and unpretentious man. I am certain that was the main reason why the Lord chose him for such an important ministry. Father knew the glory belonged to Jesus and nobody else. He was so conscious about this fact that he always referred to himself as "The donkey of the Lord," the one who had to carry Him to His people like the donkey that carried Jesus on the day He entered triumphantly in Jerusalem a week before His Passion.

Luckily for me, Tampa was the first time in a series of opportunities to meet Fr. Tardif on upcoming retreats during the following years. In all those different occasions I was able to see him in my own town, Miami. One of the greatest gifts God had regaled me with and certainly one that I will always be grateful for.

When I finished getting acquainted with Father's life and works, I pondered on my own experience. I was still sick but the retreat had definitely touched me at my deepest core. I felt that my rancor and bitterness had been replaced by a calm acceptance and forgiveness. I could never change my past or the unfair circumstances life had dealt, but I certainly could switch to a more positive attitude and outlook. I could certainly start using a more expectant faith in the power of God and finally I decided right then, that no matter how many people had hurt me, rejected me and offended me in the past, there was somebody to whom I really mattered as a human being and as a woman; somebody who cared deeply and forever about me and that was Jesus Christ.

I felt loved and that was all that matter.

CHAPTER 10

❋

FASTING MARATHON

The following day found me still with a pounding headache, sprawled all day long on my sofa with a blue ice-bag over my head. When mom came back from work, she handed me the mail and to my astonishment I saw three missives addressed to me. The physicians I had previously contacted about my condition had all graciously responded me.

The US Surgeon General Office offered to examine me in their Maryland headquarters free of charge provided that my primary physician referred me as "patient suffering from an ailment of unknown etiology (cause)." The drawback was that as their patient I needed to be willing to submit to all tests that they deemed necessary to reach a correct diagnosis. In other words, I needed to be willing to be "the classical guinea pig" which sincerely I did not mind at all along as the results were encouraging.

The second letter was from the California endocrinologist. He too, was inclined to accept me as his patient and perform the insulinoma test.

The proverbial "third time is the charm" actually became the third letter *was* the charm. Dr. Neil Wilson, an endocrinologist from Emory University was also eager to rule out the possibility of an insulinoma tumor in my pancreas. Given my precarious economic situation, he was willing to waive his professional fees.

Regrettably, Dr. Wilson had no jurisdiction over hospital policies. In order to be admitted for the 72 hours test I needed to pay up front $3,500.00 to Emory.

After a careful evaluation of the best prospect for my exam I chose Atlanta. It was closer to Florida than the other two locations, Dr. Wilson was keen to relinquish his fees, and finally my mother had a couple of old Cuban friends who lived in Atlanta who were more than delighted to have me as a guest in their home for as long as it was necessary.

There were yet two issues to be resolved before I could board a plane to Atlanta. I needed somebody to travel and stay with me in the hospital and even a more pressing issue was the amount of money I was expected to pay at the Hospital Admissions Office upon my arrival. Blanca took it upon herself to help me one more time and be with me throughout my new challenge. She was truly a compassionate, caring soul. Her actions spoke louder than her words. Another friend of mine, Martha, one of the few who had not deserted me during my three-long year ordeal with vertigo, came up with a brilliant idea to raise the funds needed for the hospital and the airfares. She and her husband approached a local Cuban Radio Station manager, and explained my case. The manager took compassion of me and set up a Radio Marathon immediately to appeal to the Miami community to make donations for my cause. The response was overwhelming. In the end we collected the needed funds to afford Blanca's and my airplane tickets, the hospital fees and even Dr. Wilson's. I am forever indebted to all the magnanimous souls who made my medical consultations in Atlanta possible. After all arrangements were finalized, almost two months had passed since my return from Tampa. I left for Emory Hospital in late November 1989.

The wheels of the American Airlines aircraft gained velocity as the jet was ready to take off from the Miami Airport tarmac. The dichotomy of both my excitement and apprehension inside the plane were intense to say the least. Looking out the window at the vast blue sky made feel smile and rejoice. Thousands of feet up in the air, above solid ground I felt an exhilarating freedom I have not felt for a long time. For a brief moment, I closed my eyes and delved into a wonderful dream. *I* was the accredited pilot. I had absolute control of the aircraft, my life and the lives of the passengers.

Power, control, autonomy. Long-lost treasures that I still craved to gain back. I was too young to be disheartened. I wanted it all; a career, a husband and children. Atlanta was my next ray of hope to get me one step closer to my dream. My wandering thoughts stopped. My apprehension waned. Neither the altitude, nor the change in barometric pressure had brought any drastic changes to my ears. I was still in a low-level dizzy state, just as I was before my departure. The flight did not aggravate my condition. I finally allowed myself to enjoy the rest of it.

The Atlanta bone-chilly weather in late November took me aback at the airport exit. In spite of my ankle-long, suede skirt, my mid-calf black leather boots, my white thick cable turtleneck, and my long wool navy coat complemented by same color, faux-leather gloves, I was shivering. Twenty-five degrees Fahrenheit proved to be too much of a draft for a tropical girl like me.

After a 45 minute's ride in a local cab, we finally stopped at our hosts' house. Enrique and Connie, my mother's friends, were already waiting for us. It was passed eight o'clock. After a warm, delicious bowl of homemade chicken soup and some oven-fresh French bread we were shown to our guest bedroom. The crackling fire in the living room and the heater in the rest of the old brick house kept us very comfortable. We slept throughout the night.

Next morning, Enrique drove us to Emory University/ Hospital building. Once we signed up at the Admissions office, we were shown to our own private hospital bedroom where the insulinoma test was to be conducted. Blanca would stay with me during the whole time. She would not have it any other way. In a few minutes, Dr. Wilson made his entrance. He was a man with a slim body structure, of average height and a premature platinum hair neatly swept to the back.

Dr. Wilson did the preliminary check up and right then Blanca interrupted him and told him that she had been praying for him during the whole trip. She had asked the Lord to guide him and enlighten him so he could determine the real cause of all my symptoms. At that point, Dr. Wilson asked me very gently,

"Would you like me to pray with you right now?

I earnestly nodded my head in agreement.

Dr. Wilson was not a Catholic but he was a Protestant. It did not matter at all. We all prayed to the same God, Jesus. He asked for guidance and implored the Holy Spirit to lead him throughout the discernment of my illness' roots. He said,

"If this illness is within my specialty, please Lord let me know so and let me treat it accordingly; if it's not within my scope, guide me to the right specialist."

When the prayer ended, Dr. Wilson proceeded to explain the whole 72-hour procedure to us. A rigorous fasting had to be established under strict medical supervision. Water and black coffee, emphasis on black, were the only beverages allowed to enter my body. Food was absolutely banned. Every 2 or 3 hours blood was to be collected from my veins to measure my insulin, glucose and C-peptide serum (blood) values.

At the end of the 72 hours fast a glucose cutoff point of 45 mg/dl or less plus high values of insulin and C-peptide would establish the indisputable presence of an insulinoma tumor in my pancreas. In order to avoid neuroglycopenic symptoms (the human brain obtains the energy it needs from glucose. When glucose levels drop to very low levels the person experiences mental fog or confusion, can't talk or act normally. Those are neuroglycopenic symptoms) Blanca was instructed to check for my mental status every so often. Simple tests like counting from ten to one in the right order, remembering a list of words and simple math problems were crucial to ensure that my blood sugar levels had not dropped to a life-threatening level. Needless to say, that my friend took her assignment very seriously until the end of the fasting.

A few minutes later a platinum-blonde nurse came to the room and applied a tourniquet to my arm, found a good vein to stick and with great precision applied the vacutainer or tube holder, secured the loose tube attached to it, and with one quick movement, inserted a fine needle in my arm. The red-stopper test tube started to fill slowly with the bright-colored fluid. It was the first needle in a long series of drawn blood samples.

The first 24 hours of the assay I tried to stay as calm as possible. I was talkative and pacing up and down the hospital corridors in my mint-green, long, flannel robe. By hour 32, I had a throbbing, splitting headache that landed me in a sulking mood and forced me to lie down. My energy was almost non-existent. Undoubtedly, my glucose levels were in a steep decline. The fierce hunger transformed me into a hostile monster. I was angry at the whole world and the stupid test in particular.

By the third day of fasting, I hardly opened up my eyes. Headache still lingered around and so did my piercing hunger. By then, I was resigned like a powerless sheep to my circumstances. I just started counting the minutes until my torture was finally over!

I reached hour 72. Hooray! I was salivating, savoring the basted turkey with cranberry sauce and the mashed potatoes with yams on the side. It was Thanksgiving Day! My elation was short-lived though. Dr. Wilson came into my room and abruptly addressed me,

"Mercedes, I need you to be fasting for two more hours. I need to perform a glucagon test to rule out an insulinoma tumor for certain,"

I stared daggers at him and complied. Time passed slowly. More blood drawings. I sustained more pain. My arm looked like a colander at the end of the assay but finally it was over and I was able to devour my "sumptuous banquet." It was the best Thanksgiving dinner I ever had in my life! I thanked God whole heartedly for my feast. It was delectable!

I finished my meal, closed my eyes and lowered my bed to relax for awhile. Three hours later, Dr. Wilson woke me up from my stupor bursting the latest news. I did not have an insulinoma. I, indeed, had idiopathic hypoglycemia but not tumor. After seventy two hours of fasting, my glucose level was below 42mg/dl but my insulin and C-peptide levels remained low enough to substantiate the ruling out of a tumor in my pancreas.

I gazed intensely at Dr. Wilson and literally I had a meltdown in front of him. I let it all out amid a torrent of tears and almost inaudible whispers. I told him how I was secretly hoping for him to inform that I had a tumor, even a cancerous one, that uncertainty was killing me, that I was back to square one, horribly sick and no diagnosis; that all I wanted was a name, the name of my enemy so I could battle him in the open, just a chance to have a fair opportunity to fight whatever it was that was consuming my life and robbing me the opportunity of having a normal youth. I told him that hypoglycemia was not the cause of my horrible vertigo, that a simple diet comprised of complex carbohydrates and some proteins every three hours would take care of it and that finally, the name "idiopathic" was indeed a very idiotic term that the medical community always used whenever they did not have the slightest idea of what in the world was wrong with a patient, that it was such a stupid term that it felt like an unpardonable insult to a patient's intelligence.

Dr. Wilson understood my frustration. He nodded his head in a sympathetic gesture.

"Mercedes, I have given ample thought to your symptoms. Tomorrow, you will see two specialists here in our facility; a psychologist and an otolaryngologist. I have no doubt that the root of your illness resides in one of those two areas. I am very sorry that you feel so discouraged and disappointed. Keep your faith up please. God will provide us with the right answer to this puzzle. In the meantime, try to get a good night rest".

Softly sniffling I bid the good doctor good night, turned off the lights above my head and closed my eyes. Blanca did not utter a single word but I heard her soft prayers in the silence of the room. The next morning I was carefully evaluated by Emory's clinic psychologist. His diagnosis? I had to keep searching for an answer somewhere else. "My physical symptoms were absolutely real; they were not in my head. I was *not* a nutcase after all."

Right after, I was introduced to Dr. Tom Turner. He was an otolaryngologist, a member of the Emory's staff. He listened carefully to my story and assured me that I suffered from Meniere's disease. To validate his assessment, he took me to a sound-proof room where a technician invited me to sit in a very comfortable black-leather recliner. Dr. Turner left the room and the technician placed a set of headphones over my ears, attached some electrodes to my head, turned off the lights and advised me not to make a sound or a movement for the next 45 minutes. In spite of the incessant, loud tapping in my ears, I managed to relax and complete the test.

The test confirmed the diagnosis.

"Here, Dr. Turner said while extending me a filled prescription. This is Hismanal, it's an anti-histaminic medication. It's the latest used to treat Meniere in our patients."

"How long do I need to take it?"

"For the rest of your life, he replied."

One more time I doubted the efficacy of the prescribed treatment and one more time I was absolutely proven wrong. In a rare illness like Meniere's you make a lot of mistakes along the way. It's inevitable. Blanca and I returned to our host's house to pack our suitcases and rest before our trip back to Miami. The next day, we said our goodbyes, thanked Enrique and Connie for their hospitality and boarded a cab to the Atlanta airport.

Case is solved. I finally got a name for this monster but . . . now what; will Hismanal put an end to my misery once and for all or is it another unsuccessful treatment?

CHAPTER 11

※

AMAZING RECOVERY

One pill at bedtime. Another pill the next day. And another one and . . . in a matter of a few days my eyes were filled with glee; it was a new whole world for me after three long years of sustained suffering. My heart rejoiced as I started a very slow pathway to my rehabilitation; my welcome back into a more normal world. Hismanal proved to be up to the task; a miracle pill for me indeed.

The terrible loneliness that consumed me for the past three years yielded to a new world of friendships, accomplishments, a new whole feeling of worthiness, and personal value that viciously, Meniere had taken away. As it is common in most severe chronic illness, isolation and seclusion from the rest of the world had taken a great toll on my psyche. I could not be thankful enough for escaping the grips of my physical separation from the rest of society. Loneliness is the greatest adversary of incapacitated human beings, who are often relegated to a state of inertia while the rest of the world keeps pursuing their regular activities.

Through a swift series of events, my life turned around for the best. I started to participate as an active member of my prayer group's activities again; sometimes assuming a position of service. We met every Wednesday to study the Scriptures, to praise God and to pray for the intentions of all our members. Every Friday we met at Carlos and Sarah's home to pray the rosary and to coordinate the meals we would serve to homeless on Sunday.

Saturday mornings were reserved for cleaning our houses, grocery shopping, running errands, and the like. In the evenings, we all attended Mass at Our Lady of the Divine Providence Church. After the religious service was over we all went to a nearby restaurant to share a fraternal meal and socialize with each other. Early Sunday mornings were spent in front of a stove, cooking huge pots of beef stew or any other type of meat, white rice and soup complemented with buns and a fresh salad. We had an assembly line at Sarah's home. Once the women finished the cooking and the packaging of the meals, the men were in charge of driving to the poorest neighborhoods in Miami and distributing the individual meals to all the homeless who wanted to receive a hot meal. It was an arduous labor; but we did it with great love.

It was my way to return to mankind the appreciation I felt for my amazing recovery. You might attribute my recovery to God's divine intervention or simply well educated, knowledgeable and compassionate physicians. It is your prerogative but it truly does not matter. In my mind, all events were finely orchestrated by a supreme being, my God and My Lord. There were no "coincidences" here; He was in charge of all the doctors, medicines, friends and prayers on my behalf. Anything and everything that had a pivotal role in my recuperation.

Very important events developed in the following weeks after my return from Atlanta. I tried to keep my weekly visits to Judith, but inevitably all my new activities found me falling behind scheduled appointments with my therapist. Eventually, Judith had to discontinue my sessions altogether. She needed me to see her on a regular basis to give her therapy a chance to work. I didn't have time for that commitment anymore. In the end it did not matter.

After a year of psychological therapy my vertigo had not subsided. Hismanal was the pill doing the trick for me. Obviously, my illness had a physical origin, not a psychological one.

The month of December finally arrived and I find myself enjoying my favorite season of the year even though in Miami the weather is as torrid as ever and the warm weather can obliterate the fact that winter has officially started in the rest of the country. Christmas' eve 1989 became a very special date for me. The prior two years I had spent my Christmas celebrations secluded at home and our traditional Cuban holiday meal went literally "down the drain". I was elated to finally be able to embrace the Christmas festivities without any incapacitating symptoms.

From our mother country, Spain, all Hispanic countries have inherited the custom of celebrating the Birth of Jesus at a midnight Mass, very well known in Spanish as "Misa de Gallo." Its literal translation is "Rooster's Mass." It is my favorite Mass of the year, always preceded by beautiful carols. December 24th, 1989 I had dinner at home and dressed appropriately to attend Mass at midnight accompanied by my mother, our Asian friend and Blanca. At the last minute, Blanca had another commitment and called me to apologize for not being able to attend with us to St. Agatha's church. We understood.

After Mass concluded, I walked up to the Nativity scene at the front of the building. I looked at the tender scene of Mother and Child and from the core of my inner being I pleaded,

"Mother please, I beg you. By next Christmas let me hold a baby of my own in my arms."
I blew a kiss to Baby Jesus and returned to my friend's car.
Silly goose, you are not dating a man, you are not engaged; don't you think that you are asking too much of The Virgin Mary

to intercede for that kind of miracle. One year. One year to find a boyfriend-fiancée-prospective husband-wedding ceremony and nine months of a gestation period. You are praying for the impossible! Are you out of your freaking mind? I scoffed and laughed at myself.

New Years' Eve 1989, Carlos and Sarah invited the whole group to an end-of-the-year party in their house. It was a Sunday. I woke up early in the morning and got ready for Mass. My Asian friend picked me up and we drove all the way to Broward County to hear Mass at St. Isidro's Church; the same church where Blanca took me before our beach outing. We came back to Miami early afternoon and agreed to meet at 9:00 p.m. to go together to the party.

I was thrilled. I hadn't been to a party in ages. I was surrounded by my new friends, enjoying fine food and of course, Latin music. The party was really animated; many couples were dancing to the tunes of popular songs of all times, contemporary and not so contemporary; actually, some of them were Latin oldies. I observed everybody joyfully twirling around from my seat.

I wanted to be part of the action, too. I was the only woman beside the golden-age ladies, who had not stepped up to the dancing floor. Luis Carlos, a young guy from our group who had been dancing with his wife for quite a while, started to ask me insistently to be his partner.

God, I want to. I want to be normal like every other girl my age. But I am scared. I am terrified.

Luis Carlos' perseverance paid off. Finally, I left him grab my waist with his right hand and his left one locked up mine. My left arm was gently landed over his shoulder. Cheers and clapping surrounded us. Everybody knew about my struggle with vertigo. Everybody knew I was wondering how in the world I would dare to turn, swing, sway and rock while following the music rhythm. I knew perfectly well that Luis Carlos' interest in me was solely to encourage me to start living again; no fears, no limitations, no vertigo allowed.

At first, I was a rigid stick that hardly moved. Then, a tap left on the first beat.

Oooh pinch me, somebody pinch me; A step forward on the same foot. *I am dancing.* A rock back to the right, a twirl and . . . *It's real, I am doing it!* I laughed, I smiled; another twirl, my hips swung left to right, forward and backward; I thanked God. *I am free of vertigo. It's over.*

Even if I wasn't back to a hundred percent my old healthy self, I was clearly heading in the right path at the speed of light.

CHAPTER 12

❀

ONE HUNDRED AND EIGHTY DEGREES

The dress was lay down on my bed as I was about to try it on for the millionth time the day before my wedding. I looked at the stream of pearls flowing down on a cascade from the high collared neck. It was a truly majestic adornment. I admired the long cathedral train displaying a fine embroidered Chantilly lace work. I delighted my eyes on the fine crystal beadings adorning the fitted Basque waistline and the long puffy sleeves with their satin bow attached to the hem. A royal garment. Wasn't that how all women think they deserve to be treated on the day of their marriage; like a true queen from our fantasy-filled heads since our earliest entry into "a girl's world"?

Reality checks in many of us much later, but for that night I allowed myself to be fully engaged in the same sweet dream that millions of young ladies before me and after me have dreamt. (I am still an optimist who believes marriage does work for some women . . . and some men of course). I filled out the tub with scented bubbles and turned on my cassette player.(How strange does that sound, right? No Ipods or Mp3's, another era!) Sweet and sensuous, Barry Manilow's melodies reached out my ears. I turned off the lights, lit up three lavender candles, covered my eyelids with cotton balls saturated in cold water; I coated my face in one of those popular cucumber masks of the eighties and submerged myself into the tub. Ahhh, I felt so relaxed!

After a restful soak, I found myself popping a colorful EBULLIENT bubble. I blew up another one. I yet chased a third one that proved to be as hard-headed as a typical teenager and refused to dissolve under my breath. How many joyful bubbles had I popped up in the span of the past 11 months? Quite a few I admitted to myself.

In January, my Asian friend—yes, the one whom I found so short for me when I met him—and I started dating seriously. Religious and community service were then tightly intertwined with our romance. Next month, the Social Security Administration office (SSA) sent me a letter that conveyed the most awaited news, "Notice of Favorable Decision". After three years of a long-standing battle, a process of appeal, denial and an official hearing process before a handicapped judge, all of my efforts had finally paid off. I was granted SSI (Supplemental Security Income) plus the much needed Medicaid and Medicaid plans to cover all my medical and pharmaceutical expenses. Dr. Wilson's assertion of a poor prognosis due to a suspected Meniere's disease had favorably tipped the scale in my favor. I was forever indebted to him. As it is customary in very rare diseases, especially in the case of Meniere's patients; it is very difficult to be granted a disability status by SSA; especially if you are a young person in the prime of life as I happened to be. As I pictured in my mind the difficult battle I had recently won, I burst out a bluish-purple bubble with exhilaration.

A playful bubble stopped right on the tip of my nose. That one was for the next victory I had attained during my impressive recovery. Within days of my SSA's disability status approval, I started working as a part-time lab technologist at two different medical offices. One was an oncologist's practice. I was in charge of performing CEA (Carcinogenic Embryonic Antigen) assays to monitor the response of cancer patients to their chemotherapy and/or radiation treatments. My other job was in a General Practitioner's office. My laboratory duty in this other practice was to perform all routine chemical blood tests on all patients. I smiled at the vanishing mixture of soap and water right in front of my eyes. Love and youth are a very powerful combination. I felt on cloud nine. I was on top of the world, ready to enjoy myself the new chapter of my life I was about to begin.

The ceremony was very simple, yet extremely emotional. As Wagner's wedding March began its solemn accords while I walked down St. Louis Catholic Church's aisle clinging to my brother's arm in a sublime state of delirium I gazed at the faces of all my guests. Streaks ran profusely on some of them, yet others bore a grinning smile to express their profound admiration and happiness sentiments. I smiled back as well.

My husband and I spent our first night together as spouses at a wedding suite in the sumptuous Mayfair Hotel located in Coconut Grove. The next day we flew to St. Marteen Island located in the north Caribbean Sea. St. Marteen is a gorgeous, little, enchanted island with superb white sand beaches and scenic hills. It is the smallest land mass in the world shared by two nations; Holland and France. We arrived at the Juliana Airport on the Dutch side of the island late in the evening. Although it was the beginning of December, it was as hot as any summer day in Miami. That's St. Marteen's tropical climate; bright, sunny and sizzling heat all year long.

We stayed in a water-front fourth floor apartment with the most incredible imaginable view of the Caribbean Sea from our balcony, courtesy of a friend who happened to be the CEO of the luxurious resort. An extravagant champagne bottle, a fine confectionary box of chocolates and a tropical fruit basket were some of the amenities we enjoyed during our visit.

In the middle of the week, the hotel administration organized a "beach picnic" at sunset. Wearing my ocean-blue swimsuit and a black pareo, I enjoyed the gracious ebony-skinned chef who wore a stark white apron and supervised the fragrant barbecue stations all the while portraying a wide smile and dancing cheerfully to the rhythm of "soca," a very popular and cheerfully-contagious music of the Caribbean islands.

Around midnight, just when I was about to retire to my room, a lady holding her coconut-leaf sombrero with one hand grabbed a microphone with her other one. It was time for the customary raffle that our hotel management staff had arranged for all of its guests. Upon arriving at the party earlier in the afternoon, I had received a numbered ticket. I turned around and looked at the yellow piece of construction paper in the palm of my hand with black numbers printed on it. One number was called; it wasn't mine. Then the next number was shouted and bingo! I was the lucky recipient of a very pleasant prize. I won a long-day trip to the renowned neighboring paradise island of Anguilla.

The next day I woke up earlier than usual and donned my swimsuit, my dark sunglasses and all the sunscreen I could gather. Before closing the suite-apartment door I double checked my box of Dramamine pills. They were secured in my straw tote. I felt relieved. We boarded a small inflatable raft that carried us to an indulging cruiser with abundant space for fifty plus passengers, most of them couples like us, to make our voyage a memorable one. Anguilla proved to be one of the most breathtaking beaches I had ever seen in my entire life; an endless stretch of white-powdery sand with a giant pool of amazingly turquoise clear water and indigo sky. The yacht moored about a mile from the shoreline. Tourists who desired to explore the fringe of coral reefs surrounding the island had the opportunity to enjoy snorkeling in Anguilla's transparent waters.

We spent the whole day virtually alone, in this mostly desolated island, lolling in the sun, swimming in the warm waters and listening to the birds sing. *I immersed myself in my three favorite "S's"; sea, sand and solitude.* We had a delicious meal of French quiche, tropical fruits, crisp salads and garlic potatoes, all prepared fresh by the experienced local crew chef. On our way back, the wind filled the mainsail, the yacht glided effortlessly over the waves, occasionally hitting some rough spots and interrupting the non-stressful motion of the vessel. I let the gentle breeze caress my face while admiring the astonishing red-orange spectrum of a beautifully colored sunset.

I made it. I survived the complete voyage without a single vertigo attack; I did not even feel lightheaded. Yes, I have been set free. Thank you, Lord. My life has finally turned around a hundred and eighty-degrees.

CHAPTER 13

❈

WISH GRANTED ONCE, TWICE, THREE TIMES OVER

"Wake up sleepy head, Moms are not supposed to sleep that much!" Debbie's voice sounded maliciously playful at the other end of the receiver.

Waaaaait, what did you just call me? I exclaimed trying to prop myself up on my bed with one arm, while holding the phone with the other one.

"You heard me Mercy; you are going to be a MOM. Congratulations!"

"Debbie, are you sure. Are you kidding me? Please don't joke about this."
"I am not joking sweetie. Your test came back positive."

Debbie was the red-haired-high-spirited-thirty-something employee hired by my oncologist chief as his secretary. Just three days before I got her call, I had been prescribed a very strong oral antibiotic for some kind of infection I can't exactly recall now. Just to play it safe, I had asked a co-worker to draw my blood and sent it out to a general lab to be tested for a quantitative serum HCG (pregnancy) test. It was the end of April 1991. I had been trying to conceive a baby since my wedding night. Four months later, my wish had finally been granted.

I looked up at the ceiling in my bedroom and thanked Mary. On Christmas' Eve of 1989 I had asked Our Mother to allow me to hold a baby of my own by next December. I had put Her on the spot with my presumptuous petition. However, in the span of a year and a half, I had dated a man, become engaged, married him and finally conceived a new life in my womb. It was clearly much more than I could expect in such a short time.

Thank you Mother. Thank you, Lord. I know that there are many women who desire to be mothers and they just can't for different reasons. I have been blessed beyond words.

My joyous motherly feelings were very soon to be shadowed by old-time detested companions; nausea and vomiting. As soon as I reached my sixth week of pregnancy, the upsurge of progesterone hormone in my body and the growing fetus in my womb became totally incompatible. The term "morning sickness" was awkwardly alien to me. My "sickness" was morning-afternoon-evening-non-stop sickness. Once again, I found myself "hugging" the toilet as an estranged husband who after long years of his departure, suddenly, decides to return home and settle comfortably in his old lodgings.

In my favor, I have to admit that not even once during those horrible first 16 weeks of continuous vomiting I had a single Meniere's attack. I had stopped Hismanal "cold turkey" right after my pregnancy was confirmed. Once my first four months of gestation were completed "the estranged husband" hit the road again. Good riddance! The rest of my gestation was uneventful except for my swollen legs and ankles; courtesy of a congenital, extremely rare condition named Klippel—Trenaunay syndrome that kept me home-bound-feet-elevated until the birth of my son. Understandably, I also had to bid farewell to both my part-time jobs.

On January 16ᵗʰ of year 1992 I went to bed at midnight. About two hours later I woke up and went into my kitchen to grab a bite. As I struggled to ascend the stair cases of my two-story townhouse to climb back into bed, my water broke. I looked at the fine fluid strip on the stairs carpet and I knew it was time to call my doc. By 6:00 am I reached the Doctor's Hospital in the city of Coral Gables. I was rushed into a delivery suite equipped with an ample bathtub to facilitate the most comfortable natural delivery possible. (Yes, those were times when you had all those little luxuries during your delivery hospital stay. I even had a lobster dinner the day after my delivery, a sorrowful difference with the current sate of health care affairs in our country nowadays).

By 10:00 am, my cervix was fully dilated but my son was as "high as the sky" in my womb. Exhausted from all the pushing and the unbearable contractions my doctor, Raymond, (a distant cousin) decided to waste no more time and proceed with an emergency C-section delivery. Oh the naiveté of first-time mothers! With each new contraction my resolve to have a "natural delivery" diminished; every new painful wave left me wrung out and desperately grasping for air. I was so terrified my heart would succumb to so much pain. When I was finally taken to the ER and had my first shot of epidural, I just wanted to embrace and kiss the anesthesiologist to let him know that he was the greatest hero in all of mankind history. I couldn't believe that I was so adamant in my decision to have a natural birth when I could have been spared from so many hours of agony. That was a mistake I swore right then would never happen again.

After all pre-op steps, surgery commenced. In a little while I felt some pressure and tugging in my abdomen. A few minutes later I heard a strong cry and after a few more minutes of waiting I finally caught a glimpse of my new-born child, a very healthy nine and half pounds-Asian-baby boy with his small head crowned with very dark hair. Well, his head was not so small; actually, it was much bigger than 'average' babies' heads. That was the reason why I could not have a natural delivery to begin with but it did not matter; after all, my baby was not deformed, his APGAR score was really high, everything was perfect. I named him Adrian Jesus.

When Adrian was five-months-old, I was hired as a Medical Technologist at the University of Miami Diabetes Research Institute (DRI). It was a full-time position. Two important events took place while I was an employee at the Diabetes Institute. One of them was grim news, the other one was a genuine blessing. A few months onto my new job, I went for a routine check-up with the Head of the Otolaryngology Department. To my astonishment, the hearing in my right ear had deteriorated considerably. The doctor was highly alarmed. He ordered an MRI on the spot. To my relief, there was not a trace of an acoustic neuroma (ear tumor). Nevertheless, the loss of hearing was a herald of true Meniere's symptomatology; if there was any doubt before about the true nature of my illness, my hearing impairment dispelled it all.

At the DRI, I met this very tall (one inch taller than I), slim, vivacious-hard-worker nurse named Desiree. From the time we met, we had a tacit understanding that there was a great chemistry between both of us. Three years my junior, Desi was married and had a little boy just like me. As time went on, we started sharing lunches and rides in the Metrorail system at the end of our work days.

Desi and I had a lot in common. We both loved our jobs, we liked to read the same kind of books; we also shared a deep love for our churches. We became fast friends. In time, we disclosed to each other the increasingly persistent feeling that had hit us both simultaneously; we both wanted to have another child, a girl to be more specific. I remember with crystal clarity going to the mall and losing myself in front of white satiny, toddler dresses with ruffled under pants and their matching headbands; the perfect outfit for a Baptism. For the life of me, I could not understand why if I was already a mother I had this gnawing desire pulling inside myself every day but that's just the way it was. Desi felt it, too. Every month we drew each other's blood and I tested it for a sign of a new life inside our wombs. Each month when the tests came back negative, we cried for a while, we held each other tightly and whispered, next time. It was our secret and our obsession.

Luck reached Desi's door first. When her baby shower was held at the DRI doctor's lounge, I tried to join the rest of our co-workers. I was stopped cold on my tracks at the entrance. I visualized the pink balloons, the pink ribbons, the pink cake icing. I knew that Desi was going to have a baby girl. However, I could not fathom that I was going to have a meltdown at the sight of the glowing new mom and her rosy celebration. I turned back on my heels and left. Next time I saw Desi it was at Jackson's maternity ward. She was holding her bundle of joy on her breasts. I felt extremely happy for her and undeniably sad for myself. Unbeknownst to me I was already expecting.

My second pregnancy's first weeks were unbearably tough. Nauseas and retching were more intense than in my previous one. This time around, Raymond had to order home medical care. A competent nurse, Lil, was arranged to come by my house every 72 hours to hydrate me with IV's. It was a rough, hard-hitting deal. My fragile veins could not stand the nightly movement of my arms. The IV needle always slipped out of place. My hand and arms were swollen and red. It hurt badly but I had to wait until the third day for the arrival of Lil. She was an angel; she had been through a horrible pregnancy herself and understood me completely. She encouraged me to endure it all with the reassurance that the pain was absolutely worthy and it would eventually go away.

Nevertheless, the vomiting was continuous; I could hardly retain anything in my stomach, ergo my sugar levels went really low; that was enough to ensue the onset of migraine headaches which were a constant part of my life by then. Raymond was reluctant to allow any pain relievers; not even an Advil so the baby would not suffer any damage. One day in particular, the pain was excruciating, I had endured it for hours in a row. My stomach's muscles hurt badly from so much regurgitating. My head felt like it was about to explode. I called Sarah in desperation. Her response was,

"Don't be afraid, I'll send Loti over right away".

Loti was a very timid, quiet, sweet lady. She was Sarah's right hand in the affairs of our prayer group, and a woman with a solid life of prayer. A grandmother and mother herself, she sympathized with my predicament. Loti bent over my bed and started praising our Lord. Immediately, she reached out for her Holy Water bottle, sprinkled me with it, and laid her hands on my head. I felt a crack. In the fraction of a second, my migraine pain that had lasted for several hours in a row was gone. I cried out of happiness. I cried out of relief. I cried out of thankfulness.

We mothers endure any hardship conceivable and inconceivable for the sake of our offspring from the very beginning of conception until we draw our last breath. Very slowly and very painfully I was beginning to grasp this concept. I was acing my course in Motherhood. Deep down inside, however, I felt this anger raging its rightful course. Why on Earth, on this rich, industrialized country there hadn't been a solid research to study a safe relief for pregnant women suffering from such a very common malady as migraines? Was my doctor really up to date on the last research about this topic? Was he really informed? Had I made a wise decision by choosing Raymond as my OB/GYN specialist one more time? All these questions revolved in my mind over and over. I would not find the answers until much later, unfortunately.

Gestation's sixteenth week arrived and with it the most anxiously anticipated respite. My "estranged husband" left for good once again; I was liberated from vomiting and free to enjoy the rest of a healthy pregnancy. I had left the DRI post as soon as nausea started never to return. Being a full-time mom became my priority. Incredibly, in the midst of my sustained stress during those tormenting four first months of my baby's development, Meniere was still in remission. By week number twenty I had my routine ultrasound. I was ecstatic, looking intensively at the monitor screen while listening to the strong heartbeat of my baby I knew at once. I was carrying a girl, my precious baby, my most awaited princess.

When my lovely angel girl turned two years-old, we arranged for a small celebration in our townhouse. Mercy asked me for a jolly ice-cream chocolate cake in the shape of a bright-yellow-Smiley-Happy Face. Yep, at that tender age my lovely girl could express herself fluently. She already knew what she wanted in life and of course she got it. The day of the party as I held Mercy in my arms for a snapshot, I knew something funny was going on inside my body; a sort of a familiar feeling. The next day I waited anxiously for the test result . . . one more time and one more time the plastic stick showed up a pink band, absolutely, positively the color of my favorite ice-cream flavor, strawberry.

Oh, oh, wait a second. This is a mistake, God. My family is complete, see? We have dad, mom, a boy and a girl; even numbers, not oddities here. We are perfect.

Really, Mercy? You are funny. Oh, girl, you definitely want to see me laugh, don't you?
Go ahead, tell me you have plans and I'll laugh my head off.
Oh, what's the use? You always win Master.

Susan Marie was born eight months later. By far, hers was the most difficult of my three pregnancies. Vomiting was continuous, unrelenting. I could not hold any food. My fragile veins were all literally exploded from so many needles. I was constantly in and out of the hospital in an attempt to keep me hydrated but in terms of medications for vomiting or migraine headaches I knew the drill; I got none. The baby's safety came first. There was this time when I had to endure a migraine headache for more than 24 hours along with the vomiting. Raymond did not prescribe any meds for the BRUTAL HEADACHE; instead he summoned a neurologist to my room. I can't remember his name but I will never forget that he ordered 100 mgs. of Demerol every four hours immediately. In his own words, "the migraine cycle" had to be broken STAT (at once). It turns out that Demerol had been proved safe to be used during pregnancies. To this day I have never forgiven Raymond for letting me go through hell during those interminable 24 hours.

The day came when it was impossible to keep me on IV's. I was not getting any nutrients at all. Whatever reserves there were in my body, my baby was getting them all. The prognosis was dire. It was a Friday morning. Raymond told my husband that as a medical professional, he could not do anything else for me. We had to wait until next Monday to decide if I could survive on my own or if an emergency abortion was needed in order to preserve my life. I was by far, Ray's most severe pregnancy case in his 25 years of practice. I suffered from Hypermesis Gravidarum (excessive vomiting) and as it was the norm with the rest of all the other rare illnesses in my life, (Meniere's and my Klippel-Trenaunay syndrome) only 0.3 to 2% of pregnant women suffer from this condition.

To my detriment, in 1997, the anti-emetic (anti-vomiting) drugs that are available today did not exist. Raymond entertained the idea of having a portal system fitted into my neck to feed me; but my veins were too thin for the required needle gauge. My fetus and I needed a sound nutritional support and we could have none. I was exhausted, I did not want to live anymore; I gave up on whatever little food I was getting at the time. Why did it matter if everything I ate ended up in a basin anyway?

That unforgettable Friday, after listening to Raymond breaking the dim news to my husband I heard a male voice in the hospital hall. The voice was talking about the Holy Spirit. I knew it had to belong to a man of the cloth. Fr. Joe Fischwick, the hospital chaplain, came into my room at once when I called out for him. A soon as he got acquainted with my situation, he started praying for me. He left me a rosary and kept coming back everyday to pray for me, to anoint me with the sacrament of the sick and to encourage me not to give up any hopes about my baby. It was a time of desperation and many more tears but by week sixteen, "the odious, estranged husband" left me for good and Susan Marie was born by a C-section delivery; a healthy-eight-and-three quarter-pound-baby girl with a faint cry and the most beautiful Asian face I had ever seen in any newborn. It was much later that I found out how many nights in the very early hours of the morning, Fr. Joe kneeled down by his bed to intercede for my Susie. My second precious princess could have been born with severe damage to her brain or her small body. Instead I got regaled with a beautiful baby, both physically and spiritually. To my delight, in due time, Susan proved to be as exceptionally gifted as both of her siblings.

Susan had an ample vocabulary by the time she reached her eighth month of life. By age two, she had learned the alphabet, the numbers, and a myriad of different colors. At four, she was reading Dr. Seuss' books. From that time on, she became an avid reader. By the time she was in first grade, she started writing her first draft of a "mystery novel". By fourth grade she had completed her first story and started working on her second one. In fact, it was Susan's creative endeavor that gave me the confidence and the much needed insight to work on my own book. Susan's IQ is extremely high. Her intellectual qualifications are simply astonishing. To this day I look at her and as I feel tears welling up in my eyes, I keep calling her silently "my miracle baby." As traumatic as Susie's pregnancy was, Meniere was still in remission. I know I could not have survived such a brutal pregnancy and vertigo at the same time. I was blessed beyond words.

CHAPTER 14

❈

"LONG LIVE REMISSION"

There followed many good years. Years settled into the routine of a busy-stay-at-home-mother of three little children—and a husband always occupied with his charts of cash flow accounts receivable and payables. Years of rosy cheeks and feverish foreheads. Years spent equally in claustrophobic doctors' waiting rooms and in playgrounds, the zoo, museums, the complex swimming pool and the local sunny beaches. Years of insatiable exploring, tumbling, insecure first steps, diaper bags and strollers sight-seeing around the neighborhood. I miss dearly all those years that went by so quickly. I truly enjoyed the nights spent "camping" in my bedroom surrounded by my "Asian troop" listening attentively to scary stories and funny ones, putting on little skits and playing new games all products of our active imaginations. I miss bonding with my three angels. It's a stage all mothers go through. We are seized by severe lack of sleep; the days seem endless, time is standing still and you wait anxiously until you are able to finally bond with your bed on a more normal schedule, a slight resemblance of life before . . .

In spite of it all, time flies. One day you look back and your little ones are not so little anymore. One by one, they start their own journey by venturing into that intriguing place called "school." From there on, homework, school projects and extracurricular activities are all part of your children's daily routine. You learn to start letting go. Little by little, until one day it's all about,

"Hi, mom. Can I go out mom?

I need a book for an assignment. Yes, today mom."

Well, at least that's the phase I find myself right now but behold; I know what fate is awaiting me in a few more years. One after the other one, all of my children would leave the nest. It is a painful experience that my older friends have endured with great bravery and resignation, biting their lips while the tears flow freely down their faces. Nevertheless, all of them have survived the transitional stage from industrious worker bees always stifling their own needs to tend to everybody else to a more relaxed and yes, solitary lifestyle something more along the line of a queen bee.

At any rate, for approximately the next ten years my life resembled the typical life of any other suburban mother raising her young offspring. Meniere was absent from my hectic life and, honest to God, I did not think about it anymore. It was deeply buried in the back of my mind; camouflaged by my frenzied lifestyle. My God-given-right to dream about pursuing a PH. D in Microbiology/ Immunology was magically transformed by unprecedented and unforeseen circumstances into a new scholarly degree. A degree for which there are no universities or post-graduate study centers in the whole wide world that bestow my newly acquired diploma. In the years subsequent to 1992 I graduated Suma-cum-laude in the most honorable degree of all times: a Doctorate in B-a-b-y-o-l-o-g-y; which has been and always will be the greatest accomplishment of my humble life on this planet.

One of the biggest delights kids experience every year in Miami from March to mid-April is the Miami-Dade County Youth Fair better known as "The Fair." In March of year 2000, I took all my kids to enjoy the traditional monster roller coasters rides, the haunted houses and the kiddies' rides for the youngest ones. As I sat on the benches in the early evening waiting for the Circus to start, munching on a warm elephant ear, I felt a horrible pang in my belly. I could not move. I was struck by fear and pain. I remained seated for over an hour and when the show ended, so did our stay at the fair for that year. The pain diminished somewhat but persisted for two more days and then it all went away the same way it had arrived.

Later in the year, exactly on Thanksgiving Day, the pain returned in full force. By then, I felt a great lump right below my navel. I was transported to the nearest ER. Immediately, I had a stomach x-ray series the results of which were dismissed as a simple case of the stomach flu virus.

"But Doc, what about the "ball" I feel below my navel?"

"Oh, that's just a scar from your previous three C-sections."

"But how come I have never felt it before?"

"Now, you never looked for it before, did you?" And with that impressive insight I was sent back home.

The next day I had to be rushed back to a different ER. This time, luckily for me my "ball' was a strangled umbilical hernia about to rupture at any given moment. The surgery was scheduled STAT. The surgery itself was not a big deal but my migraines became a horrible nightmare. As soon as I was put on a fast as a pre-op measure, my glucose went down and my migraines flared. Any migraine sufferer knows from experience that as soon as a headache starts, you need to counteract it with your medicine or the price you pay is an unendurable pain accompanied by nausea and vomiting. Hospital personnel did not seem to have any migraine sufferer on board that day. From the time I complained about my migraine until I finally received Imitrex (my migraine medication), more than three hours passed by. The nurse, following due protocol, had to call the doctor in charge of my case who happened to be at a meeting. When he finally returned the nurse call, the hospital pharmacy did not have Imitrex in stock, so they had to order it form their supply company. At that point, I totally regretted my decision to relinquish all my personal medications to comply with hospital policies.

By then, I was a total mess. I threw up violently until only bile remained in my belly. My pain was excruciating and I got a cocktail of Toradol, Imitrex and Compazine drugs, in a vain attempt to stop my symptoms.

Let's just say that the "cocktail" was not as tasteful as a Blue-Coconut-Margarita. It did not agree with my metabolism at all. I had a severe allergic reaction. What was supposed to be a very simple surgical procedure became a horror. I required general anesthesia to compensate for my allergic reaction instead of the standard epidural. Finally, two days after my operation I was discharged from the hospital with a scar in "my tummy," a trophy to prove that I was right all along and a bottle of Percocet to pacify the post-op pain in my abdomen.

Two days later I tried to do some laundry. My two older kids were gone to school. Only Susan, three at the time stayed with me.
"Susie please bend down and pass me those clothes from the dryer; yeah, like that baby."

Susie stretched out her very small hands and started handing me the unfolded clothes. I tried to focus on the task at hand regardless of my mid-section pain and then the weirdest feeling in my life struck me out. My legs didn't move. I couldn't stand-up, walk or lie down. All I could manage was to sit on the floor, in spite of the brutal abdominal pain and I let the tears flow freely. My hands started shaking; I had these tremors. I had no idea why.
"What's wrong with me?"

My baby looked at me in disbelief. Mommy was fine one minute, now mommy is sick?

"It hurts mommy?"

"It hurts but it's not my wound baby." That's all I managed to express.

It is my soul that it is hurting. I am overcome with fear, great fear. I am losing my mind. Oh dear God, I am losing my mind," I told myself silently.

Looking retrospectively, it all seems utterly funny now; although there is nothing really funny when you are embedded in a serious depression crisis.

What I found amusing was my primary doctor's reaction the very next day when my husband took me to see him and my own ignorance

"Doc, am I losing "it? Am I insane?"

"Of course not, and the whole concept of you being able to pose that question is the best indication that you are "not losing it." You are just suffering from "chronic depression and anxiety." Just so you know, depression and anxiety go hand in hand; they are the proverbial two sides of the same coin. We need to treat both at the same time with one medication, sort of kill two birds with one stone. I SHOULD WARN YOU THOUGH; IT IS GOING TO TAKE AT LEAST SIX WEEKS BEFORE YOU FEEL TRUE RELIEF FROM YOUR SYMPTOMS. THAT IS THE WAY ANTI-DEPRESSANTS WORK, VERY SLOWLY. C'MON CHICA, SMILE AND GET OUT OF THE HOUSE, GO ON AND HAVE SOME FUN. GET SOME FRESH AIR. HERE IS A REFERRAL TO SEE A PSYCHIATRIST. THE MEDICATION WILL STABILIZE YOU." My doc assured me with an ample smile.

In spite of his reassurance, I left the office sobbing, nagged by doubts. Just the mere thought of my three little angels, ages eight, five and two-and-a half at the time made my eyes inundated with continuously flowing tears. To this day, I don't know the reason why but then again, nothing makes much sense when you suffer from depression. Depression goes a long way back in the history of medicine although it was not until very recently that the current term was adopted to identify this ailment. Many theories have been used to explain what causes it but there is not a general consensus among the medical community. Some theories run from genetics to the environment, to a chemical imbalance in the brain; henceforth, the therapeutic benefit of current pharmaceuticals. Was there any inkling in my life as to what awaited me before I came out of my surgery? No, there was none. To date, I am still questioning myself how big a role my hernia surgery's mishap played in the onset of my gloomy moods.

The first anti-depressant tablet I was prescribed was Paxil, a medication that belong to the newer class of antidepressants named SSRI (selective serotonin reuptake inhibitor). It did not agree with me. It increased my weight significantly. I had to discontinue it. Then, I was paired with another drug, Zoloft (sertraline), and that was the guy for the job. Nine years later, I am still taking it daily, although in a smaller dose.

CHAPTER 15

❊

COLOR MY WORLD BLUE, SO I CAN CHASE AWAY "THE BLUES"

The medical community has established that in order to be diagnosed with major or chronic depression, you need to exhibit at least five of the following symptoms; depressed mood, loss of interest in pleasurable activities, insomnia or excessive sleeping, fatigue nearly every day, feelings of worthlessness or excessive guilt, agitation or psychomotor retardation (inability to move), overeating or eating too little, and recurrent thoughts of death or suicide. I must have displayed some of these symptoms to my primary physician but for some reason the most vivid ones in my mind were my constant crying, my inability to put a stop to the flood of my tears, and my nervousness with its constant palpitations and wringing of my hands.

I am not qualified to diagnose or give medical advice regarding either Meniere or depression on these pages. By sharing my personal story with all of you, I strive to give you an insight of my own struggles as these illnesses struck me one after the other. My main desire is to provide you with some tools as to what worked for me, and what didn't. If these "tips" and "experiences" seem too subjective and mainly geared towards women is because they certainly are. They are *my own experiences dealing with depression.* I am a woman and a stay-at home-mom. However, most of my tips can be implemented by men as well as working women.

Over the next few days following my first depression bout, I could simply not be in charge of my life. My tremors and tachycardia were so bothersome that I could not think about anything else. I could not execute any of my domestic tasks anymore; not even the simplest ones. Nevertheless, I had three small kids who needed my care.

The first sign of relief came to my doorsteps disguised under the appearance of a Cuban old lady named Angelina. My first reaction when I learned her age was,

"No, I don't want an old lady in my house. She won't be capacitated to help me out with chores and the children. I don't even want to meet her.

My husband insisted. I said, "Fine, I'll see her and get rid of her at once."

I went downstairs, teary eyed, fatigued, trembling and met this stout, uneducated, cheerful lady portraying an ample smile on her round face.

We clicked instantly. Leave it to country people to be healthy and strong as a horse! Boy, Angelina could take on any young woman any time or day. She set to her tasks at once, my husband left for work and I stayed behind licking my own wounds, curled up on the living room sofa, just giving some instructions here and there.

Angelina was the hardest working housekeeper. She cooked, cleaned, did the laundry, vacuumed and did I mention cook? I'd ask her for any of my favorite Cuban/ Spanish recipes and presto. Little by little I started to trust her, to depend on her; she gave me a great security. She was not a regular maid; she was my lifeline at the time. She was awesome with the kids and the quality that I admired her for the most was her great sense of humor. When I was buried deep in my saddest feelings, whether valid or not, she would always manage to make me smile or she would carry on herself further and she would spontaneously resort to all sorts of antics. Many times, she made me forget entirely about my new affliction. It was just her personality. Although three out of her four children remained in Cuba at the time; a typical Cuban dilemma since the arrival of Castro to power—the separation of close families for years to come, in many instances forever—Angelina managed to carry on with a light heart. I could never thank her enough for her invaluable help when the "blues" stormed unexpectedly.

Henceforth, my first practical advice to depressed people, especially busy wives and/ or mothers is to SCREAM FOR HELP. This is the right time to make your burdens as light as possible. First, and foremost, you need to seek medical treatment. In this slump of an economy, if you have health insurance, congratulations; half of the deal has been made. If not, seek out any local mental health facilities that might treat you for free or charge on a sliding scale based on your household income. A word of caution: Depression can suck in so much of your energy that you might feel like picking up your cell or surfing the web for referrals is an insurmountable task. If that is the case, ask your spouse, partner, parents, siblings, friends or a trustworthy co-worker to make that phone call or that web search for you; it can save your life, literally.

Second advice. Recruit some outside help, at least until your meds start kicking in and you feel you can manage on your own. If your mom is alive, healthy and very close, enlist her as your primary assistant. If not, perhaps a very dear sister might work wonders for you if she is able to lend you a hand or both. You need all the help you can get at this stage. If not, a true friend, who is willing to go that extra mile for you, might be the best solution. If nothing of this sort is available but you have a solid financial situation, it might be well spent money to hire some help around the house, although it can be expensive. I did not have a "solid financial situation," neither did I have a close relative to lend me a hand. We had no other alternatives than to finance all external household help.

In any case, this temporary help may give you the most needed respite you need to find your way around depression and/or anxiety. This extra help would be a much needed break until your doctors, medications and *you* can figure out the best course of treatment in your case; a break that will lead to positive results.

You need to relax as much as possible. You need to learn all you can about this illness, especially if you have never met anybody who suffers from it. The more information you gather about it the best prepared you will be to fight it back. Search the web for information regarding you condition. Borrow books on the topic from your library. Ask your physician all pertinent questions regarding your condition.

I was truly blessed by the support of a lady I had met at my new parish prayer group and whom to this date I have the honor to call, "my mom." Olga came to my rescue when I was first hit with depression like she had done it two years earlier when I was pregnant with Susie and vomiting constantly. Olga had a petite, slim physique and was sweet as a pie. She was well into her seventies and was fit and full of energy as any young woman. She did help the children after Angelina left at five in the afternoons. From babysitting to picking up meds at the pharmacy there was no task that Olguita, as I affectionately call her, would not do for me and my family.

Although I am grateful for all of her efforts, what I appreciated the most was *her company.* I was too fragile during that period in my life, too scared and too vulnerable to stay by myself. I remember with crystal clarity one day I could not hold it myself. I was too anxious, too nervous to be alone with the children. I was exhausted from fighting my palpitations and lack of breath. I was horrified at the prospect of Olguita leaving me alone. I also needed to sleep. Xanax, (my anti-anxiety medication) had worn me out and I needed to rest desperately.

I begged Olga to sit down on the rocking chair at the foot of my bed and keep me company while I slept. She nodded in agreement. I doubted her. She assured me she would not leave me until I had rested and she did. She stayed with me for the next two hours. God bless her! To somebody who has never been caught up in the throes of depression or anxiety it makes absolutely no sense to picture a thirty-year-something-old apparently healthy woman to be frightened of staying at her safe home in the company of her three healthy children by herself. But this is exactly what anxiety can do to you; therefore, you need to counterattack with all resources available. Don't be shy about it: ask for help.

A word of caution here: Depression can distort the way you envision your world, the way you envision reality. Too many people suffer from recurrent suicidal thoughts to ignore this destructive, way too common depression symptom. If you feel you are going down that tricky, slippery slope, send a holler and get some help. Call a hot line number, a friend, a family member, your pastor or priest but please talk to somebody. Your life is precious to God and to your family even if it doesn't seem like it when you are burdened by the gloom and doom of depression. Suicides do not only destroy depressed people's lives but also the lives of their loved ones. Never, ever assume that your loved ones would be better-off without you. It is a dreadful deception that depression plays on your afflicted mind.

Third advice. It might seem contradictory but . . . get closer to your children and let their love soothes your raw nerves.

Children are amazing creatures who can either make you pull out your hair in downright despair or can get you in a state of wild elation. In most instances, they make you laugh hysterically. I, personally, chose to bond, to get closer to my children in a supreme effort to calm myself and to assure them that my condition has not taken mommy's love away from them. Here is a brief list of some activities I embraced at that time with my young kids. We watched Disney movies together. For some reason those family movies put me in a serene state like no other activity could. After all, there was no real, menacing violence in *Little Mermaid* or *Toy Story*. We would also go to the library and sit down there for hours to read except with brief intermissions for bathroom breaks and to savor a hot-dog and a soda.

Even Susie, the youngest one in a stroller behaved perfectly well. I sat her on my lap and read some books to her. I thank God for blessing me with children who are avid readers. I think those were the only times when my children would not fuss and behave like angelic creatures. Other calming activities were coloring books or pictures with Crayolas and water colors. None of my children became a Picasso (well, actually my oldest daughter has surprised us all with her amazing high school charcoal portraits) but we enjoyed those times together when the little ones' imagination knew no boundaries and I felt an awesome connection with my offspring. Whether singing, dancing, doing puzzles, reading or watching movies, find activities where you can spend glorious time with your little ones and give a vacation to your stressed out nervous system. Don't be afraid to embrace the company of your little ones. Another word of caution here: the only exception to this advice is if you are suffering from post-partum depression or a severe depression that you are considering ending your life and the lives of your children so they don't have to suffer in this world alone, without their mother. In that case, it is imperative to seek medical treatment and to be SUPERVISED AT ALL TIMES. If you need to remove yourself from your children's company until you are back on your feet, please do so. It does not mean that you are a "bad mother." On the contrary, it says so much about your character by being able to take responsible steps to ensure your children's safety.

Warning!!! If your progeny are teenagers, well, we have a different entire game here. Then, it's better to explain them as calm as possible all the details about your illness so they don't get anxious and . . . keep your distance from them when they don't seem to be on their most civilized mood!

Fourth advice. Pleasurable experiences.

Stress has no place in anybody's life, much less in a depressed or anxious patient. Learn to avoid anything that might trigger sad or dramatic experiences. Override television news. Most of them are about real tragedies anyway. You are not being a selfish human being here. You are just protecting yourself so you can be a healthy and productive member of society. In due time, you will be in a much safer place psychologically to cope with world tragedies.

For the same reason, avoid relatives or friends who can bring down your spirit. You all know the type; those people who are always sicker than you are, more burdened than you are, lonelier, poorer, in an economic and social dump, always angry, gossiping, criticizing and finding faults in every single human being. Sorry, but you need to get better yourself in order to help other distressed people. This is no time to assume Mother Theresa's role no matter how laudable it might be.

This is a time of your life when you need to live in a cotton-candy-colored-dream-world. In my own experience, I have noticed that something as simple as surrounding myself by my favorite colors, mostly aqua, teal and rosy pink would put a smile on my face. As simple as that! That is why I decided to paint my girls' bedroom with those particular colors and to dress myself with those hues. Decoration has always been one of my favorite activities. Even though, I could not afford to hire a renowned decorator (sorry David Bromstad) and pay a visit to Ethan Allen's furniture store (always a dream of mine) I could spare a few bucks on Lowe's or Home Depot's paint cans and give my home a "face-lift" with my favorite colors. Try it yourself. The key here is to do something that brings pleasure to you and your senses and keeps you busy at the same time. Of course, this advice also applies to any other hobby or interest you deeply enjoy. Fishing, playing a sport, gardening, exercising at a gym or at home, whether in the company of friends or alone, reading, playing an instrument, listening to your favorite songs, painting, sewing or writing are some of the activities people in general enjoy the most. Don't let depression win the battle. Fight it with all your power and paint your world blue (or red, or orange or whatever color you fancy) to chase away the "blues."

Along with exercise and the rest of the pleasurable activities I have mentioned, I think that massage deserves a special place of honor in the battle against depression. In the days that followed my surprising diagnosis, I noticed that a back-rub and a foot massage worked wonders to place me in a state of great relaxation. If I coupled them with a pleasant aromatic candle (vanilla and lavender being my favorite scents for the bedroom, apple-cinnamon for the kitchen) and soothing music I felt as if I were in seventh heaven. If you are blessed enough to afford a spa or a professional massage, center take advantage of it. Spas offer different packages and deals that cover a vast array of massages alone or in combination with facials, manicures, pedicures and other pampering services; yes, they do offer services to both females and males. In most cities, you can subscribe to www.livingsocial.com. The site offers one fantastic deal everyday with discounts of up to 90% at local restaurants, bars, spas, theaters and more. If you are even luckier enough to have somebody to help you in this department in the privacy of your own home, embrace wholeheartedly the "help." If not, there are many different massage apparatus that come in different sizes in today's market. They are not necessarily expensive, and like I said they would work wonders for you. Give them a try! LADIES DON'T BE SURPRISED IF YOUR HUSBAND OR PARTNER IS THE MASSEUSE AND ONE THING LEADS TO ANOTHER . . .

CHAPTER 16

⟳

MORE USEFUL ADVICE

Fifth advice. "What do friends and Religion have in common?

When most people talk about depression boosters and anti-anxiety relaxation techniques they never fail to mention all the different kinds of yoga and meditation so common nowadays in our culture. I have to apologize sincerely to you my readers because yoga, (none of its varieties) or any other Asian sort of meditation has ever made it to my "to do" lists in my ongoing battle against my condition. Whether it is that I have always lacked time-energy-resources—and good health (can you imagine me trying to strike a tree or a lotus pose while seized by dizziness and disequilibrium?) or just simply because the concept is as foreign to me as the Australian aborigines; I had never entertained the famous yoga suggestion as a relaxation technique.

That does not mean that I haven't or don't practice meditation and relaxation at all. Relaxation can be summarized as calmness of the heart, soul, body and mind. When you are "anxious or panicked," your nervous system becomes activated in a "fight or flight" response. Your heart rate increases, so does your blood pressure, your palms sweat, breathing becomes more rapid (hyperventilating) and so on. As a consequence, your pain level intensifies. Relaxation techniques should be practiced on a daily basis to make you feel calmer, experience less pain, lower your heart rate, improve your breathing, and lower your blood pressure.

The following relaxation technique is very simple to achieve and it might do wonders for you. Just set aside a quiet time, possibly at the same time everyday.

1) Lie down or just sit up with your spine straight.
2) Close your eyes and gently place your hands on your abdomen or by your side. (If room is too bright you might use an eye mask). Feel free to put on an instrumental CD.
3) Start breathing through your nose.
4) Push the abdomen outward S-L-O-W-L-Y as you exhale.
5) Close your eyes. Visualize your feet. Inhale, exhale, and let them RELAX. Don't move your feet anymore.
6) Now, visualize your legs. Repeat process. Inhale, exhale, relax. Don't move them anymore.
7) Repeat the same process with all of your organs and body parts, your hips, your torso, your ribs your stomach, your arms, your neck and your head, back and sides alike.
8) Think about your favorite places; it might be a childhood place or somewhere you would love to be right now. Be an active part of the scene! Smell the flowers, listen to the sound of the waves crashing through the shore, gaze at the shining stars on a clear night summer sky; whatever calms you and makes you feel pleased.
9) I have different images that I use when I relax. A summer day, young girls cloaked in pastel dresses running freely through a meadow totally covered with wild bright colored flowers, a sunset by the beach, a sparkling sea and a refreshing breeze caressing my face, a cold, winter day and the warmth of a fire log, the sweet aroma of pine and a hot cup of cocoa amid my friends' laughter and so many more! You just need to find what works out best for you!

I have established from the beginning of this book that I was raised in the Catholic Church and I am still a practicing Catholic.

Nevertheless, it is my intention to reach patients from all cultures and different religious backgrounds throughout these pages; however, if I want to do a genuine and honest job I have to recount this tale from my own perspective.

"Meditation" for a Catholic is very different from the concept according to some other religions, where "meditation" involves a quieting of the mind and all senses. Catholic meditation is quite the opposite; it is a very active undertaking (not physically active but mentally). For all obvious reasons, the best way to meditate is to choose a quiet place where you know you won't be disturbed by anybody, neither children nor nagging husbands. Turn off the TV, the phone, the Blackberry, the I-Pod, and laptop. Seclude yourself from all distractions. Once you are isolated from physical intrusions, adopt a posture that it is comfortable but not too comfortable so you don't end up in a deep slumber. There are basically three steps in Catholic meditation.

The first step is to place yourself in God's presence. Close your eyes and think of yourself being accompanied by God. Just call on his name several times until you bring Him into your mind. This might take a while but it is crucial to do so before you start meditating. You'll know you are there when you feel your heartbeat slowing down and you are enveloped by a serene peaceful feeling.

The second step is the meditation itself. Imagine a scene from the Scriptures.

(Even if you are not Judeo-Christian, you might be inclined to approach something that you have never attempted before in your spiritual life) Think about what the environment might have looked like. Picture the place and the people, what they look like, what they are doing.

Imagine sounds, words people are saying. Imagine yourself interacting with the people there. If it's a scene from the Gospels, which character would you like to play? If Jesus is present what would you say to Him? How do you think He would respond to you?

You might stay there as long as you want or need to. The last step is to give thanks to God for helping you to meditate. Perhaps He has revealed a word of comfort you never expected to hear from Him. Or a precise course of action is firmly revealed to you. You won't necessarily hear His voice but a persistent thought may come across your mind and you know it could only come from Him.

I have practiced this type of meditation mostly at home, and retreats (especially silent retreats), where I am not allowed to talk to anyone but God (either by protocol or by my own decision) After listening to different reflections throughout the length of the retreat (if at home I might choose to listen to a CD with a recorded reflection or read a Scripture passage) I engage in this type of meditation step-by-step. It is a practice that has helped me tremendously to relax and change the perspective on the outlook of my life.

I can vouch for the same outcome about prayer in all of its types and forms, whether communal or in the solitude of my bedroom. My prayer group has been a constant support in my life and a great source of strength when my depression set in for the first time. At the beginning of my diagnosis, things shifted tremendously. I became a passive member of my group instead of an active one like I was used to but I made the commitment to attend every week to the meetings even if somebody had to drag me there. The effort was so worth it. Back in those days I did not want to sing and praise God as I was accustomed. My depressed mood kept erroneously signaling me that all past joy I had experienced in praising God had been robbed from me forever.

In as much as depression did not allow me to find joy or pleasure in my group as before, God still did *find joy in seeing her daughter praising Him.* Jesus is never depressed. I am the one who had changed. He never does. That was a very reassuring fact, although, I could not absorbed that truth at the time.

See, it does not matter which religion you practice. What really does matter it is THAT FAITH IS AN ANCHOR that keeps you in touch with a reality behind your comprehension; that you are God's creation and He will never abandon you. FAITH is a greater force than you are; a force, a God that you cannot see with your human eyes but you can *feel and perceive at all times. A God that is much alive and loves you so much more. He will do anything to bring you out of your turmoil and misery. A God who directs your steps so no harm might come to you. You are safe in His arms. A God who would be your friend forever.*

Since we are brushing up on the subject of friends, I mentioned before the pivotal role my friend Olga played during my initial depression crisis. Thank God her friendship has continued flourishing up to this date. Olga was not the only friend who provided me with a heartfelt support.

Elizabeth, Eli, my friend from my early teenage years back in Cuba and her family was a strong, reliable backbone (and still is, thank God) which allowed me to cope with my condition without falling apart.

I take the time now emphasizing the importance of belonging to a group that gives you a sense of community. My own mother was very ill, end-stage liver cirrhosis at the time I developed depression. In fact, she just went to meet her creator four months after my first bout. My mother-in-law had passed away the previous year. The rest of my beloved relatives who stayed back in my country were deceased, too. I had no family to rely upon. I was a stay-at-home wife and mother; I had no co-workers to lend me a shoulder to lean on but my prayer group was a solid network of support when I thought I couldn't go on any further.

So you see, God is our friend but usually, I mean except in a very few rare instances, He does not reveal himself to us in person, He does not materialize in our earthly world; nevertheless, He tends to our needs and in most instances to accomplish this mission He uses "angels" to assists us. Those "earthly" angels are called "friends."

By experience I know that when you are deeply submerged in the throes of depression you don't want to do absolutely ANYTHING. You don't want to see absolutely ANYBODY. You just want to curl up in bed, pull up the covers over your head and let the house burn down. But that is not the kind of life that God envisioned for you when He created you. If you don't have any close relatives or if they are old and in frail health, your FRIENDS are the army God sends you to pull you out of the pit you have fallen into.

I know it takes a steel will to take the firsts step to come out of your shell of isolation and sadness. But, for you own sake make the effort to extend your hands to that army of soldiers called friends to allow them to pull you out of that black hole you have slid into and bring you up to the surface.

How can you do that? You might ask yourselves. Well, you know all those times your cell is playing whatever tune you have chosen and you stare up at the name, sigh, and put the cell right down on the coffee table totally discouraged? Don't do it. You might let it ring once or twice but if by the third time your cell is still vibrating and playing "You should have put a ring on it" or your home phone is ringing off the hook, ANSWER IT.

Your caller ID is telling your friend Alice is worried sick about you, TALK TO HER. ALLOW YOUR SOMBER VOICE TO SAY HELLO, slip into a pair of slacks or leggings, tie up some comfort sneakers, don on a sweater or a top tank if you live in torrid Miami, (won't hurt if you comb your hair and apply some lipstick) and head out for the door with your friend Alice. A cup of coffee or some tea if you are too jittery, a veggie pizza slice and some fresh fruit at a quiet shop or restaurant will invigorate you and provide you with a different outlook. Yes, I know you don't feel like going anywhere because what's the point anyway if you are depressed?

Don't worry. This is not about what you believe when you are feeling all down; it's about all the things you need to do until you become your old self. Frankly, friends are the best force in the world to help you get there.

A walk in the park, a manicure and pedicure (you might throw in a blow dry if your budget allows it, too), some shopping (yes, window shopping counts too) in the company of a dear friend will definitely gives you a boost until the veil of depression has been lifted up for good. Trust me, eventually it will. What about my male readers?

Well, men by their social upbringing are not as partial as women to sharing their emotional side with their friends. That is okay. As I mentioned previously, an invitation to a basketball game, a fishing trip, engaging in any other type of activity or sport is a great achievement, both for you and for the friend who managed to drag you out of your cave. If you have a woman in your life who loves you for who you really are confide in her. Ask her to be supportive until you get out of the abyss. Just be truthful and considerate of her limitations and right to live her own balanced life. Seek medical help please!

The idea as you might imagine is to get out of the house, to feel alive, to look at your surroundings, enjoy nature, allow the sea breeze caress your face, watch children play and laugh. Remember that life goes on like before. Yes, you have encountered an obstacle in your path, you feel sad, discouraged beyond words but give some time to your meds, doctors and lifestyle changes and you will overcome this trial. Depression has no cure but it is a very successfully, treatable condition.

Put a smile on your face, even if you don't feel like it; fake it. Trust God and trust your friends; they are somehow connected to work together to let you remember that your life is invaluable. Gradually, you will start feeling better and when you reach that stage, be grateful and return the favor by helping out others in need. There are a myriad of charities and volunteer opportunities. You will be in a win-win position; you will feel much better about yourself both physically and emotionally all the while reaching out to other human beings in a more precarious situation than yours.

I, for one, am grateful that even in the midst of my depression I never abandoned my prayer group and vice versa. I allowed my group to pamper and coddled me all I needed it but as soon as my medications started doing their job I went back to work in my church according to the best of my abilities.

CHAPTER 17

❦

A SUMMARY OF DEPRESSION BOOSTERS

-Rest all you need. If you are having trouble sleeping, ask your doctor to evaluate your condition to determine if you might benefit from a sleeping pill. Lack of sleep worsens your depression at an exponential rate. In fact, I would rate it the number two trigger after stress.

-Eat a healthy, balanced diet. Cut down on fats and sugars and have more veggies, fruit and lean meat. Three good meals and two healthy snacks in between should be enough to keep you away from unwanted cravings. Being hungry or sleepy is detrimental to your condition. I need to reinforce these points.

-Stay away from alcohol and caffeine, especially if you are suffering from anxiety. Although I seldom drink alcoholic beverages myself, (imagine the combination of alcohol and Meniere); nevertheless, my physicians have always illustrated for me the devastating effect that alcoholic beverages have on depressed patients. Alcohol simply increases their depressive symptoms exponentially. (Of course I am not referring to the occasional glass of Chardonnay you might enjoy at a celebratory dinner!) The same holds true for illicit drugs. Seek professional help if you suffer from any of these lethal addictions. There are much healthier ways to cope with depression.

-Exercise regularly. As tired as you are, make a maximum effort to engage in some type of physical activity. Exercise has been proven to help counteract depression and help with sleep.

-Aim to have self-control in your life, a more positive attitude and personal success.

-Remember, work is not only a way to support yourself; it should also give purpose to your life.

-Don't be bashful about your condition; ask for help until the storm has subsided. Remember that "friends" are vital to your recovery.

-When you are depressed you derive very little enjoyment from normal, daily activities. There is no sense of pride in your achievements anymore. Your joy has been "stolen." Your insight and judgment are affected; you are incapable of functioning at work or in society. You are not longer able to make changes for the better; you are paralyzed.

If the following thoughts keep coming back to your mind

"I never do a good job."
"I am a failure."
"Things will never get better."
"It is impossible to have a better day."
Or
"Nobody loves me/ nobody gives a damn about what happens to me."

"I am positive I am a burden to my family. They will be much better off without me."

"Suicide is my only way out." "I just want to stop from hurting so much."

If you recognize yourself in this description, don't waste another minute and seek professional help.

Medication by itself does not address underlying problems behind depression, but it certainly changes your mood for the better. Why should you put your life at risk and be miserable when there is so much medical help available?

Be aware that there are certain types of depression that cannot be managed without medication. Others require medication for just a set amount of time. In any case, it is up to your psychiatrist to determine the best course of action for you. Trust your psychiatrist; follow his medical plan for you. Don't ever stop your meds without you doctor's approval. Anti-depressants CAN NOT be stopped abruptly. There are serious side-effects if you do so.

After I was diagnosed with chronic depression, nine years ago, I was never able to receive any type of psychological counseling. I did not have the time or financial resources. However, I would venture to say that most depressed patients might benefit tremendously by seeing both a psychiatrist (who is a licensed medical physician certified to provide prescriptions) and a psychologist or licensed counselor who is trained to help clients to solve negative evaluations of themselves, the world and the future. Antidepressants are the mainstay of treatment but when coupled with psychotherapy it improves the outcome considerably.

One fairly common psychological approach nowadays is CBT (Cognitive Behavioral Therapy) It aims to replace dysfunctional behaviors, thoughts or habits with a more reasonable and realistic views of one's feelings and behaviors. I emphasize that I have not received psychological counseling as part of my depression treatment but I definitely would love to have the opportunity to explore psychological counseling at this point in my life. I firmly believe that anybody who has suffered from a very traumatic event in their lives; in my specific case, sexual abuse as a child, should benefit tremendously from mental counseling. Remember that, "Scars will only remind us where we have been but they don't dictate where we are going."

Warning. Even after we recognize when our mental processes have gone awry, it might take precious time to change deep-seated behaviors and thoughts. Customarily, mental counseling is EXPENSIVE. Is it worth it though? I certainly believe so and medical statistics back up my assumption.

-Enjoy nature and the beauty of this world in general. Relax and appreciate your surroundings. Pursue you hobbies; perhaps a new one? Little things can amount to big things. Don't underestimate the power of a new lipstick shade, a new fragrance or a new book.

- Enjoy music. Relaxing music that calms down your nerves is beneficial. Happier tunes can put you in a festive mood. Music should be one of your best allies in the fight against depression.

-If you are suffering from anxiety, I strongly urge you to start each new day with a "LIST TO DO.". If you have help around the house, the burden would be eased for you. Whether you do, or not, I've found out that a piece of paper and pen at the beginning of my day helps me cope and control my anxiety very efficiently. See, the idea is to compartmentalize your day, to break down your activities into small blocks that are much easier to manage than a whole list of "priorities."

I love to think that I have become a master at my "to do lists." On one side of the paper I write down house chores I intend to achieve on a particular day. On another side I jot down my kid's activities. Errands to run? That makes it to another side of the paper. Sometimes I need two sheets of paper. Sometimes I use a small journal. It does not matter what I use for my notes as long as I use "something" as soon as I have my breakfast! As the day wears off, I scratch off my completed tasks. That gives me a tremendous sense of relief and control. Somehow, I am still in charge of my life. It is important to have order in your life and not chaos if you want to enjoy a more peaceful existence.

-Structure is fundamental to control anxiety. Plan each new day the *day before.* If you are fortunate enough to work on a daily basis, avoid chaos in the mornings. Choose your wardrobe, make-up, purse and jewelry you want to wear the night before. Prepare your lunch; make sure you have money in your wallet and gas in your car. If you have school-age children, review their assignments the night before. If they are young, prepare their uniforms and lunches as well. Plan ahead your family breakfast; all these simple measures can avert an anxiety attack in the mornings.

-Let your children come to you and enjoy them! They are not a BURDEN. They are God's more precious gift to you. Kiss them, hug them and tell them a million times how much you love them. When you do that you are "investing" in the well being of your children; you are planting seeds of love, security and encouragement in your little ones. The pay-off will go a long way. You will reap the fruits of your unconditional love in due time when they become independent, self-sufficient, mature, well-balanced, adults; with integrity. In the meantime, you will also get to experience the purest form of human love in our world, the precious love of a child.

-I emphasize once again the intrinsic value of volunteer work. Even when the walls seem to be closing up on you, there are many people out there whose lives are much worse than yours. As soon as you feel a little better, go out and offer your help to other unfortunate souls. Your body, mind and soul will be rejuvenated. You will discover a new purpose for your life. You will enrich other lives beyond words. Since my children are still young and occupy most of my time, I volunteer at my parish's children prayer group. This way, am still get to be with my kids and help my community.

-Don't harbor resentments in your heart. It will only make you feel more miserable. Perhaps those closest to you don't understand what you are going through. For your sake, don't expect them to. Let your doctors explain everything about your condition to them. Be patient and allow them to develop patience towards the new "you." Any chronic illness is bound to put strains on any family. Don't despair, your family still love you.

-You might feel anger toward God, relatives, and even yourself. Rest assured that no one is to be blamed for your condition.

-Forgive offenses for your own sake. Let go of burdens and lighten up your heart. How can you do it? Stay away from all people who have caused or might harm you and do not engage in any vengeful acts against them. Instead of cursing, blaming and planning revenge acts against your enemies pray for them, speak blessings over them and ask God to stop you from all interaction with those people. Let God be your avenger. He is a just God. Even if you are an atheist, stay away from negative thoughts and plans. Let go but do not let go of your dreams and plans for the future! You need to concentrate on what really matters to you and your family. You would also derive an inner peace that no one can steal from you. Focus on all the blessings you have in your life. Cherish them. This is a time you need to invest in yourself; physically, emotionally and spiritually. You don't need an extra burden with everything else you have to contend with.

-Set up new goals for your life even if you are too sick right now to envision them completed. A person needs to live his life pursuing one dream after another one. If you can't keep things fresh and new illusions in your heart, you soul will be like a languishing plant. I love the way the renowned world pastor Joel Osteen expresses this idea,

"When one dream dies, dream another dream."

". . . . Stir up those dreams, stir up those talents inside. Start stretching yourself. You are meant to dream and to pursue the desires God has placed in your heart."

". . . If you don't have a dream, you're not really living the way God intends. You're merely existing. Maybe at one time you had a dream, but you went through some disappointments or setbacks. Things didn't turn out the way you planned. But here's the key: when one dream dies, dream another dream."

From Daily Devotion Daily Word—We Dare To Believe website.
Daily Word from Joel Osteen, Joseph Prince, Rick Warren, Kenneth Copeland ministries.

Clinical Major Depression is certainly a setback, but don't let go of your dreams yet! Our country is going through tough times financially. We are all experiencing the effects of the economic depression; some people more severely than others. We can expect to have more people depressed as stocks plunge down, jobs disappear and retirement savings just evaporate into thin air. No matter what have caused you to fall into the claws of depression, don't give up your dreams; be ready to counterattack. Little by little you will win the battle.

I would like to add a comment or two about the ongoing economic crisis that is impacting millions of Americans. If you have been laid-off recently, and you feel discouraged please don't give up on your job search. I encourage you to read all sorts of articles about job search strategies on the web. Devise your own plan for job hunting and stick to it daily. Look for places that offer Career Orientation Seminars. For example, here in Miami, you can visit West Dade Career Center. It is a great facility that lists all job positions available in different companies, from the modest positions to the most lucrative ones. You can look it up in the web. Cyber networking is crucial in today's world. Sites such as Guerrilla Job Search and LinkedIn are crucial sites for job hunters. You may also check out Guerrilla Marketing for Job Hunters 2.0 from your library or purchase your own copy. Use your social network sites to your advantage as well. Facebook and Twitter would let know your contacts about your new endeavor. It is a new game in this tough economy. You need to revamp your job search strategies!

-Take baby steps, don't beat up yourself about all the things you are not able to do at this time. It is okay. You are focusing on recovering yourself and stabilizing your mood at this time. If you only managed to take a walk out of the house for ten solid minutes, instead of half an hour, applaud yourself. If any given day, you only manage to do some laundry, fold out the clothes and prepare peanut butter sandwiches for your kids, it's okay. You have been seriously committed to take all your meds? Give yourself a reward. You are checking into that rehab facility you have always thought you did not need it because you could control your addictions after all? Give yourself an outstanding ovation. Focus on your achievements as little as they might seem. Cast out all negative thoughts. Congratulate yourself and celebrate your accomplishments, you deserve it!

-Do practice relaxation and meditation techniques daily.

-Trust God with all you heart. He will never disappoint you. He will see you out of despair AND SET UP YOUR FEET ON SOLID GROUND.

Even if you don't believe in God, He believes in you. I encourage you to call on His name and ask Him for his help. You have nothing to lose. If you don't know how to do it, this is a very simple prayer to ask for God's divine intervention in your life,

"Dear God, I am going through a tumultuous time in my life right now. I need all the help I can get. I don't even know if I believe in you or not (or I used to believe in you and now I don't find you close to my heart like I used to) but I am asking you to help me out here. I am asking you to help me get better. I know that if you do exist you will answer my prayer. I ask you to forgive all of my sins and wrongdoings. Guide my steps to the right places. Most of all, I ask you to grant me peace. Amen."

Psalm 40.

"I waited patiently for the Lord;
And he inclined unto me
He brought me up also out from a horrible pit,
Out of the miry clay,
And set my feet upon a rock,
and established my goings.
And he hath put a new song into my mouth,
even praise unto our God:
many shall see it and fear
and shall trust into the Lord"

This is one of my favorite Psalms!

The psalmist says that all I have to do is clamor to God and wait to see how many favors He bestows upon me. He bends down to my place. He snatches me out of my horrible pit, (depression). He sets my feet upon a rock (gives me new strength where there was only desolation). He takes me into new paths, He puts a new song into my mouth (I used to complain and whine about everything wrong in my life). Now, He is showing me to appreciate all the blessings in my life: my family, job, friends, shelter, food, clothing, medications and the list goes on. I am learning to praise Him, to acknowledge His favor upon me, and to trust Him with my life because He would never let me down.

All of these practices improve quality of life of all Menierians, depressed people, chronic illnesses' sufferers and all human beings.
THEY ARE MEANT FOR EVERYBODY!

CHAPTER 18

— ✿ —

GENERAL FACTS ABOUT DEPRESSION

−**A**t its worst, depression can lead to suicide, a tragic fatality associated with the loss of 850 000 lives every year!

-According to WHO (World Health Organization) depression was the number fourth leading contributor to DALYs-the sum of years lost due to premature mortality and the years of productive life lost due to disability—in year 2000 in developed countries. By 2020, depression is expected to rank in first place, surpassing all ischemic illnesses (i.e. cardiac infarction and stroke)

-According to NIHM (National Institute for Mental Health), approximately 26.2 % of Americans ages 18 and older suffer from depression in a given year.

-One in four adults ages 18 and older suffer from a diagnosable mental disorder in a given year.

-MDD (Major Depressive Disorder-also called Unipolar depression as opposed to Bipolar depression-) is the leading cause of disability in the US for ages 15-44 in a given year.

-Median age at onset is 32; although, depression can manifest itself in young children as well as elderly.

-It is more prevalent in women than men.

-With regard to pharmaceutical treatments, there is a newer class of anti-depressants called SNRI's (serotonin-norepinephrine reuptake inhibitors). In 2004, Cymbalta (Duloxetine) was approved by the FDA (Food and Drug Administration) for the treatment of major depression. In May 2008, Pristiq (Desvenlafaxine) became available on US pharmacies. Abilify is another resource that it is recently used in addition to regular anti-depressants. These are just three examples of new medications available in the arsenal to combat depression. As with any other medical treatment you NEED TO DISCUSS WITH A QUALIFIED CLINICIAN your condition to be properly diagnosed and treated. Luckily, nowadays, doctors and patients have more resources available to them than thirty years ago.

There are several types of depression; each type exhibits both similar and unique, distinctive symptoms. Only a specialist can determine which class is affecting a particular patient. Depression in all of his scope it's a very grave affliction; I just wish to discuss two of its most critical varieties here.

According to NIMH data, PPD (Post-Partum Depression) occurs in approximately 10 to 15 percent of all pregnancies. That means approximately one out of every eight women will be affected after childbirth. About 500 000 women in the United States will suffer from PPD every year. There is a 25 percent chance of recurrence with every subsequent pregnancy. It is very important for women to realize that PPD is not a failure on their part, or their fault but it is rather a serious recognized medical illness. The symptoms are very similar to any other type of depression. No woman should suffer from this disorder and hide it for fear of the stigma attached to the condition. If you or any other woman you know exhibit symptoms of depression report them immediately to a physician. Untreated PPD can have devastating consequences.

Depression in teenagers.

If you are unsure if an adolescent in your life is suffering from depression, consider how long one or more of the following symptoms have been present, how severe they are, and how different the teen is acting from his or her usual self.

WORD OF CAUTION. If your teen starts exhibiting one or more of the listed symptoms have him drug-tested either at home or by his pediatrician. Drugs and alcohol abuse is the scourge of modern society. Depression often co-occurs with anxiety and substance abuse, with 30% of teens developing a substance abuse problem.

Signs and symptoms of depression in teens.

- Sadness
- Irritability, anger or hostility
- Tearfulness or frequent crying
- Withdrawal from friends and family
- Loss of interest in activities
- Changes in eating or sleeping habits
- Restlessness and agitation
- Feelings of worthlessness or guilt
- Loss of concentration
- Thoughts of death or suicide

Depression in teens can appear very different from depression in adults. The following symptoms are more common in teenagers than in adults:

Irritable or angry mood. Irritability, rather than sadness is often the predominant mood in teenagers.

Unexplained aches and pains. Depressed teens complain frequently about headaches and stomachaches. If a thorough physical exam does not reveal a cause, they might be due to depression.

Extreme sensitivity to criticism. Depressed teens are very sensitive to criticism, rejection and failure.

Withdrawing from *some* but not all people. While adults tend to isolate themselves when depressed, teenagers tend to keep at least some of their friendships. However, they may socialize less than before, pull away from their parents, or start hanging out with a different crowd.

Untreated teen depression can lead to:

Problems at school
Running away
Reckless behavior
Substance abuse
Low self-esteem
Eating disorders
Internet addiction
Self-injury (cutting themselves)
Violence
Suicide

If you think a teenager you know is at risk for suicide, take immediate action. Call the National Suicide Prevention Hotline at 1 800 273 TALK or CALL 911.

If you ever have had a relative or a friend who has succumbed to suicide, please do not blame yourself. If your family member or friend was receiving therapy, you tried to help in every conceivable way you knew how and in spite of it all, that person took his or her life; it is not your fault. If you have been severely affected by such a tragedy you need counseling and therapy to help you cope with your suffering. It is very important for everyone to understand that when a patient is heavily medicated, usually, he has no strength to attempt taking his own life; however, when the patient is stabilized a little bit, it is more likely that he may carry out the suicidal thoughts. In many instances, if a person has no desire to live and does not believe that life is worth the effort, he might be driven to commit such a drastic act.

CHAPTER 19

—— 🌀 ——

DEPRESSION MYTHS

There are many reasons or even combination of reasons why a person might become depressed. Traumatic life experiences such as the death of a loved one, divorce, loss of a job or home, war or being a victim of a violent crime or abuse may all contribute to the onset of depression.

When a person is a "victim" of a widely recognized traumatic event, people tend to be more lenient and understanding. When there is no such a "visible known cause" such as in the case of a brain chemical imbalance, (the most widely accepted depression cause at present) substance abuse, hidden personal dark family secrets, medications side effects or genetic predisposition among others; those less obvious or acceptable reasons might be cause to stigmatize a depression sufferer.

In many instances, people decide to suffer alone, to mask their pain and try to go on with their lives instead of reaching out for help to avoid the taboo associated with mental illness. In my own experience, I have heard my own share of sarcastic, caustic, hurtful, cruel, insensitive, tactless, and ill-informed comments such as

"But why can't you snap out it?

"You know what people say about you? They say that you are a lazy person; that's right, so lazy you are using depression as an excuse in your life."

"It's all in your mind. Why don't you shake it off for God's sake?"

"I would never take those meds you take; I have a strong will and I won't take those dangerous pills ever."

And the worst of all,

"You are crazy! You are a lunatic. You are psycho!"

If you have been a victim of these malicious accusations already,

PLEASE, DO NOT FALL INTO THAT TRAP AND DO NOT ALLOW ANYBODY TO INSULT, DEMEAN OR CRITICIZE YOU.

If you could snap out of it, if you could shake it off, wouldn't you? Nobody likes to be sick, depressed and unable to enjoy life. My reply to those people is always the same,

Do you suffer from hypertension, diabetes, arthritis or any other common disease?

Yes? Then, why don't you snap out of it?

Why don't you forsake all your pills, use your strong will and eliminate all those medications from your life?

Isn't truly amazing how people can be so ignorant as to offer those unsolicited comments to a depressed person when they would never dare suggest anybody else stop their medication or their doctor visits if they suffer from any other corporeal ailment? Most people encourage others to seek out medical help when they are certain of the illness, except if it is depression.

I truly pity ignorance, and the people who fall prey to it. But I have learned not to allow harsh comments to interfere with my resolution to seek a better life for myself. Rest assured that *you are not crazy!* I wonder, don't people realize that schizophrenic patients are so out of reality that they do not know what is going on with their own lives?

There is a huge abyss between these two completely different conditions. So, no, "you have not lost it", and do not let anybody tell you otherwise. When confronted by negative people and their negative comments, it is time to flee the scene. You need support and encouragement; you need to surround yourself with positive influences. If some people can't understand your condition, suggest to them to read about it, become better informed and until they do, stay away from them!

Unfortunately, some young patients do not escape unscathed. They endure many hurtful comments:

"Don't take anti-depressants because you'll never get admitted into an Ivy league University."

"You will be denied any type of scholarship if the university finds out about your depression."

"If you visit a psychiatrist say good-bye to any political career."
"You will never be able to climb up the corporate ladder once the administration finds out about your "blues."

What more can I say? Misunderstood, false, distorted and unenlightened statements. That's what they are.

Most reputable universities have established a whole array of counselors and professionals to help students who suffer from mental illness. It is absolutely untrue that a student would be denied acceptance, financial aid and /or any other scholastic privilege based on his status as a depression sufferer.

If anything, this subset of students would be assisted to overcome their affliction and to succeed on their future endeavors.

As far as I know, there are two very capable and valiant congressmen who have admitted publicly that they suffer from depression. None has ever been deemed incompetent as a result. More recently, celebrity Catherine Zeta Jones has publicly admitted that she suffers from Bipolar Disorder. Her famous husband's struggling battle against cancer triggered a bipolar crisis that prompted her to be admitted into a mental facility to be stabilized. Other celebrities such as Demi Lovato, Britney Spears, Demi Moore, Carrie Fischer, Brooke Shields, Anne Hathaway, Paula Deen, and Billy Joel and many more have also acknowledged they suffer from diverse mental problems such as chronic depression, bipolar depression and post-partum depression. Kudos to them for their bravery! There is no shame in recognizing when you need help. As long as a patient remains faithful to his medication regimen, responds favorably to it and remains supervised by a certified specialist, depression should not be an obstacle to reach for the stars. And this list is truly comprised of "famous stars", which are widely acclaimed, admired and loved by millions of fans. They all have managed to overcome their mental conditions and live very productive lives.

If I sound like a spokesperson and an advocate for mental illness, you are darn sure I am and a very proud one, too! When dealing with depression there is simply no space for archaic ideas and taboos. Don't waste your time blaming your DNA, upbringing, or weak personality. It is just a waste of time. We need to fight for our wellbeing and a better quality of life; discrimination and misconstrued facts have no roles in our lives.

Since this chapter is devoted to debunking depression myths, I would like to interject a clarification about one of the most misunderstood depression treatments reserved for extreme cases that do not respond to any other therapeutic intervention; ECT (Electro Convulsive Therapy). ECT is generally used in severely depressed patients for whom psychotherapy and medication have proved ineffective. It may also be considered a treatment when there is an imminent risk of suicide, because often ECT has much faster results than antidepressant remedies. ECT uses electricity to produce a brief seizure in the brain that seems to jostle it back to normal. It is widely acknowledged as the most effective weapon for treatment-resistant depression in a psychiatrist's arsenal and often the last resort.

During ECT the patient is anesthetized with an intravenous injection of a barbiturate or other anesthetic. The muscles are temporarily paralyzed with the drug succinylcholine, which prevents the violent jerking motions that used to break bones during the therapy. In bilateral ECT, electrodes are placed above each temple. In unilateral ECT, the electrodes are placed above the temple on one side of the brain and in the middle of the forehead. An electrical current is then passed through the brain, inducing a grand mal seizure.

When the patient awakens, there might be a headache, nausea, temporary confusion, and muscle stiffness. Most patients report loss of memory of events that occurred in the days, weeks, or months surrounding the ECT. Many of these memories may return although not always. Some patients have also reported that their short-term memory continues to be affected for months. Severely depressed children are also treated by ECT.

Although there is still a heated debate among the use of ECT among some opponents of the practice, it has been proven beyond doubt that electro-convulsion therapy is a powerful and highly effective weapon against the most intractable cases of major depression.

CHAPTER 20

❈

BAKER ACT, A HORRIFIC TRUE STORY

As deplorable as discrimination and taboos that surround major chronic depression are, the following case is a poignant example of why at least some people, actually, most people are very cautious before admitting any mental affliction. Although, the field of psychiatry in America has seen many reforms that allow mental patients to be treated with much more dignity and respect than in the past, unfortunately, there is still more work to be accomplished in this area.

I have decided to write this chapter as a revelation and an eye-opener regarding psychiatry, the law enforcement, depressive patients and the public in general. It is my most profound wish that the following account be publicly acknowledged to avoid a repeat of the case in point.

When I informed a very dear friend of mine that I intended to write a book about Meniere and Major Chronic Depression she asked me for a very special favor,

"Please Mercy, I beg you, tell the public my story. If I can save another victim from a recurrence of what happened to me, I will consider justice properly served." For obvious reasons, I have changed my friend's name as well as that of her husband to protect her privacy. For all purposeful intents I shall call her *Pamela*.

On November 12th, 2004, Pamela Meadow, a thirty-something, married woman with three young children went grocery shopping early in the afternoon. When she returned home from her errands, she put away her purchases, served dinner to her youngsters and retired to the bedroom. As she was resting in her bed; her husband came back from work. It was about 6:00 p.m.

Pam's husband is unfortunately, a "chronic abuser." He is an extremely manipulative and controlling man who fits the typical profile of all abusers. To her detriment, Pam did not fully realize the extent of her husband's dysfunctional character until that ominous day.

An uneven tempered man always quick to be carried away by his severe outbursts, Mr. Meadow, started lashing at and thrashing his wife on that particular Friday afternoon. Something as trivial as Pam's refusal to attend a church meeting on that specific night was enough to enrage her husband as never before.

When Pam asked her husband to leave her alone and reiterated her firm position about not going to church, Mr. Meadow went ballistic. Pam left her room and headed for the kitchen. She looked at the counter and speedily grabbed her car keys. She then announced to Mr. Meadow who was right behind her that she was going out until he calmed himself. A demon possessed Mr. Meadow at that moment. He jerked back Pam's arm, snatched the keys out of her hands and began yelling right in her face. He forestalled her from leaving.

Pam moved swiftly, grabbed her husband's car keys and made it to the garage. That sealed the deal. Mr. Meadow's controlling and abusive temperament could not allow such an insult to his person. Screaming at the top of his lungs, he grabbed Pam by the neck and threw her down on the garage floor; then, he overpowered her by putting all his weight on her. He pinioned her arms behind her back to fully immobilize her. After a struggle, Pam pretended to be calm and sat down on her living room sofa. Still in a daze, she eyed the door, surveyed the space between it and the sofa, and launched herself to the exit. It was to no avail. Pam's crazy husband got a hold of her and subdued her one more time. Pam saw her last effort to escape totally obliterated.

At that point, Pam cried and yelled and told her abuser that she was going to call the police. THOSE WERE THE MAGIC WORDS. As if propelled by a spring he jumped off her and yelled at their oldest child, who was twelve at the time.

"Son, dial 911. Tell them it's an emergency, **DO IT, NOW!!!!!**

Pam's son, as in a trance, obeyed robotically.

In a few minutes, two young police officers, one Anglo and one Hispanic arrived. They by-passed Pam and went straight to her husband. They jotted down all the malicious lies that Mr. Meadow disseminated. Pam was a depressive woman who refused to take her anti-depressive medications. He had found her in a frantic state after he came back from home and that he considered her a threat to herself and others. Could they please be sympathetic and help him? He was at his wit's end and suffering so much to see his poor wife in such a predicament. What if she would harm herself or the kids?

Not surprisingly, Mr. Meadow failed to recall that he started yelling and lashing out at his wife as soon as he came back from work, that he threw her on the garage floor and prevented her from leaving the house just because he was a controlling, manipulative, Neanderthal, deranged, abusive individual who ruled his house with an iron fist and could not tolerate "No" for an answer. He also omitted (inadvertently I am pretty sure) that the only reason he summoned the police was to save his own skin. He knew that if his wife would have called the cops herself he would have been sent down to the precinct on charges of domestic abuse. Jail time for the honorable, the admired, respected Mr. Meadow? No way; not if he could prevent it. And finally, he completely forgot to mention that Pam had never, ever stopped taking her anti-depressant medications since she was diagnosed. Somehow, he had twisted all the facts into a huge, gigantic, colossal, massive lie and he had succeeded. His falsehood had been bought by the cops unquestionably to the last detail.

One of the officers kept Pam at a considerable distance from her spouse while the other one interrogated him and her children. Pam was not allowed to speak on her behalf until Mr. Meadow was finished with his own side of the story. Then and only then was she addressed by the police.

"Maa'm do you suffer from depression?
"Yes," she replied,
"Do you take any medications for your condition?
"Yes, of course."
"Would you like to come down to our headquarters for some marital counseling?"
"Okay," Pam said reluctantly. Then, she was accompanied to the squad car. When Pam saw herself behind those divider iron bars between the back seat and the front row, an uneasy feeling invaded her. She felt like a common criminal. By then, she expressed her desire to remain at home, but her own young son, undoubtedly instructed by her father and the officers insisted that

"For her own good she should allow the good men to take her to their headquarters."

Poor kid. Little did he know what humiliation his mother was about to be submitted to and that that night incident was the beginning of the end. Marriage ceased on that night for Pam. Over. Forever.

Pam was still suspicious, but did not want to upset her boy and agreed to the ride. When the patrol car pulled over at the nearest hospital Emergency Room, Pam was immediately questioned by a nurse who started an electrocardiogram. When Pam noticed the electrodes stuck to her chest, she realized that it was all a mistake. She was not sick, she didn't need an EKG. Pam tried to get out of the gurney and leave at once. Security was summoned to her side and politely but firmly, the guard instructed her to remain calm and do as told.

"Why can't I leave? Pam replied with disbelief in her voice. I am not sick. I need to go home."

"No. Ma'am, you can't leave."
And for the very first time in her life, Pam heard the words.
"You can't leave because you are under *the Baker Act law's protection*"

Baker Act? What the heck is that? Pam struggled with the newly introduced concept. After recounting the evening's events to a long line of nurses and doctors, some of them cynical enough to laugh in front of my poor friend and some of them compassionate enough to expedite her transfer to a mental facility as required by law, Pam reluctantly decided to comply with all instructions. Her mind was fixed on only three things actually, three persons; her young children.

Pam was shuffled the next morning to a mental hospital; she was separated from her kids. Upon arrival at the psychiatric institution, she was stripped of all potential "weapons." Her clothes and bags were confiscated, and her body was submitted to a humiliating search.

She encountered the horrors of living among "real mental patients" people who exhibit a co-morbidity; that is they are either addicted to drugs or booze or both and also suffer from diverse psychiatric conditions, all of which were much more severe than my friend's properly managed chronic depression.

One elderly woman came into Pam's room and urinated on the floor while talking in a childlike voice and begging Pam to call her son to take her home. Another lady who seemed well enough, disclosed to Pam that she was schizophrenic, she kept several python snakes as pets, her daughter was bipolar and was institutionalized and oh yes, she was leaving the hospital in a few hours. Her first errand was to stop and buy some rats to feed her "babies"; poor things, nobody had fed them while she was in the hospital. Of course, she also planned to see her 'dealer' because she needed a "fix-up" right away.

One particularly handsome-young-looking guy wearing a broad smile and shaking hands with all those around him, suddenly seemed to be having a conversation with someone unseen to Pam or anybody else. When a nurse reminded him that it was just a delusion, that no demons spoke to him he replied caustically, darting fire from his eyes that "IT WAS NOT A DELUSION TO HIM! HIS DEMONS WERE REAL TO HIM!" His mouth spit hatred when he talked. Pam retreated to a corner of the community room out of more than justified fear.

At night, a roommate asked Pam to pee in a cup for her. Drug screening was the way to start the hospital daily routine. Her roommate was not qualified to submit a "clean sample." Pam refused but by then, she was horrified and wondering why on Earth, her husband had done something like this to her. Oh yes, she remembered. **Mr. Meadow was desperate to protect himself from well-deserved charges of domestic violence.** In order to do that, he fabricated a carefully woven tale. Male police officers believed it without further questioning. The same people, who had sworn to defend and protect law-abiding civilians, had let down my friend.

Her husband had taken his mask off once and for all. He had revealed who he really was to his wife. It was their fork in the road. Pam swore to herself that from then on, she would never trust him again. It was an eye-opener. Henceforth, she was alone in this world, nobody to look after her. The person whom she had trusted her to be her rock and friend to the end of her life had betrayed her, had shattered her trust and she knew he would do it again and again and again. Because that's the way abusers are. Pam would never be able to change him. She had to leave her abusive relationship. No marriage can survive abuse and betrayal.

The hospital thermostat was set up in the 40's permanently. Pam asked a nurse for seven blankets. Still, she could not sleep; she continued shivering and quivering all night long. Patients get agitated if temperatures are high. Wardens need to keep things in order as much as they can. That is why, by 6:00 am all patients have to submit a urine sample and line-up to take a cocktail of medications that calm them down, and place them in a "zombie-state", easier to manage, easier to avoid any incidents where force has to be used. Undoubtedly, chilly temperatures contribute to keep things "under control."

Pam finally met her assigned psychiatrist in the early hours of the next day. She gave him a detailed account of why she had ended up in a facility where she did not belong to in the first place. She provided her regular psychiatrist's name and telephone number. She begged the hospital psychiatrist to check with him; he had treated her for years and never, ever, had he committed her to a mental hospital.

Finally, Pam spoke her mind to this psychiatrist. She told him that her husband had her committed to avoid being sentenced himself for domestic abuse; that police enforced their rules without a second thought about who was telling the truth and who was not about their marital dispute. And lastly, she told the doc that she was at her husband's mercy from that moment on. Mr. Meadow had succeeded at getting away with his crime. Who could say he would not attempt to repeat the scam all over again?

As far as Pam was concerned, her spouse could hit her, thrash her, kick her, hurt her badly, leave her body full of bruises, and just simply summoned the police and tell them that 'his wife' did that to herself and that she needed to be in custody for her own sake and the sake of her kids and there she would be again; enclosed in a loony bin, at the most selfish, sadistic whim of her husband. She was in his hands and he knew it. To add injury to insult, the law enforcement system had failed her, completely.

The hospital psychiatrist assured Pam that that would not be the case. He, personally, would write an explanatory note on her record. Should her husband attempt to pull the same number on her, legal action would be on her side as per hospital request. Pam was grateful for the effort but still she was angry, resentful and in fear. Exhausted, she went to her home and children. None of them have been able to visit their mother while she was hospitalized. Their innocent minds could not imagine the horror that their mother had lived through because of their father's abuse.

Pam was *coerced* into admitting that hers was a voluntary admission. She was threatened to be committed for 72 hours as the law allowed it if she refused to cooperate. Eager to go back to her kids, she agreed to acquiesce to the "voluntary admission" charade, a further act of human degradation. That is how she envisioned the whole situation. Mothers go to unimagined tests for the sake of their children. She wanted to hold them and kiss them and never let them go away from her embrace again. She was released 24 hours after.

After several months of battling bureaucracy, Pam finally obtained a copy of her medical hospitalization records along with the police officer's report; it read:

"Subject was found crying hysterically (no kidding, after all the abuse she was submitted to?). Subject suffers from major chronic depression and according to her husband she refuses to take her anti-depressant medications."

That was it. No verification of the incidents occurred on that particular night. Not a shred of doubt on the officers' minds. After her release, Pam sought legal counseling from different national mental health advocate groups. She was "invited" to participate as a guest at the *Oprah Winfrey show* to relate her story nationally. Once again, Pam placed her children above herself. She declined the offer in order to protect her children from public exposure. She did not want a display of her family's grievances on national TV. Her motherly' love was put to the test one more time. *For their sake, she thought, for their sake.*

Pam's real story is an incredible example of the discrimination and marginalization to which depressed people are submitted. Although not too many patients go through this *"Cuckoo's nest"* modern version, the truth of the matter is that *depressed and mental patients in general are treated unfairly as a group* because *of prejudice and stigma.* Pam was oppressed, harassed and victimized because she suffers from depression. Had she been free of her mental condition her husband's ruse would had not prevailed so easily.

Let this be a painful lesson to all. Though likely, you will never live through her ordeal you need to know how laws might be twisted around to serve the malevolent agenda of an abusive spouse or other close relative who requests the Baker Act be applied.

The Florida Mental Health Act of 1971 is commonly known as the "Baker Act" in Florida. It was originally enacted at least in part, because of widespread instances of elder abuse, in which one or more family members would have another family member committed in order to gain control over their estate prior to their death. Once committed, it was very difficult for patients to obtain representation and they became warehoused until their death.

The Baker Act allows for both involuntary and voluntary examination. It can be initiated by judges, law enforcement officials, physicians or mental health professionals. A relative can petition admission under the law provided that the patient has a mental illness and he/ she is a danger to himself, herself, or others. Examinations may last up to 72 hours. After examination a patient might be released back to the community or placed in a mental facility for treatment.

The *Act* was named after a Florida State Representative, Maxine Baker, who had a strong interest in mental health issues, served as a Chair of House Committee on mental health, and was the bills' sponsor. The nickname of the legislation has led to the term Baker Act and "Baker Acted" as an intransitive verb for invoking the Act to force an individual's commitment.

Ironically, the same law that was enacted to protect mental patients was used to victimize my friend. Society's perception is that the "mentally ill" in general are not valuable because they can't work, are to be feared, are not worthy of respect or trust. They are seen as "different". In Pam's case, as in many other instances, this notion is absolutely false. Pam is a valid member of society who has raised three, intelligent, warm and caring children. She had never neglected her duties as a mother because of her illness; on the contrary she has been a very valiant woman who has worked very hard to overcome the obstacles of such a crushing illness.

Seven years after the infamous Baker Act incident Pam underwent, her dear son, the child who was used by his father to call the cops on his mother is showing the devastating effects of such a profound trauma. Pam's son is in desperate need of psychiatric treatment at present. However, he refuses to seek treatment mainly because he is fully aware that if he is labeled with "a mental condition," his father could pull the same deception on him as he did on his mother. What a great tragedy! Pam's Baker Act incident has claimed another victim. A young life is at stake now and there is nothing much she can do to help out her son who, understandably, does not want anybody to know about his ailment. Abusers' crimes do not end with deed. The repercussions last for years. They break down a whole family.

By sharing Pam's story, I seek to vindicate her, her family and all depressed sufferers who have been degraded and marginalized at some point in their lives because of their condition. Pam's was also a textbook domestic abuse case. In a bizarre twist, the police was initially called in at Mr. Meadow's behest. This behavior is very typical of abusers: "I am going to call the police before you do, so they believe me and don't believe you." Society needs to become more aware of the dangers to which depressed-abused women are exposed to.

CHAPTER 21

—— ✤ ——

THE TRANSITION TO THE MOST DREADED "BILATERAL" STATUS

With three young children running around our two-bedroom townhouse, up and down, side to side, left and right; our humble abode became tiny, small, and constraining to say the least. We decided to move on and move out of our complex to expand into yet another townhouse with an extra bedroom. I wanted my son to be separated from our girls. We needed the extra space.

To our dismay after a long and tiresome search we finally found a modest house to accommodate our budget. Our contentment, however, was short-lived. Our neighbors, our closest, next-door neighbors were the outcasts of our new surroundings. Two young boys who had fallen prey to drugs and an alcoholic mother who lived from her deceased's husband retirement were simply too annoying and extremely dangerous to be ignored. They would slept throughout the whole morning and by early afternoon the thuggish boys of the condominium would gather around their front entrance, sit on the family's old battered truck and start carousing. Night after night, dispersed beer cans and the residual stink of consumed weed would linger in the air and on the lawn. The noisy parties with blaring rap from two gigantic size speakers were enough to keep us awake all night long. Sleep became a precious commodity that eluded us day after day. Police squad cars were summoned on some occasions but there was nothing the officers could do about it.

Just when I was experiencing such a difficult time in my life, Igor, a dear and old friend of mine from church inherited his dad's flourishing business. He moved his family into a flamboyant new mansion secluded in a well known Miami residential area. Igor proposed we moved into his spacious four-bedroom old house with a rent to buy option agreement. I had three young kids to worry about; I did not think twice before accepting his generous offer.

Three months after I had moved into Igor's house, my friend dropped by unannounced on a Friday evening. As I finished cleaning my supper dishes, Igor entered our house and aimed straight for the kitchen. He looked tired, he pulled a chair from our old country dining set and handed me a small Tupperware container,

"Mercy, can you warm up this soup for me?"

"Of course, dear," I replied.
As I served my friend his soup, I sat down and looked at him anxiously,

"So . . . what's the big occasion that brings you into my humble home? Are you ready to discuss financial plans for the closing of our deal?"

"Mercy, have you ever heard of the term *mantle cell lymphoma?* Igor replied expressionless.

I was silent for what seemed an eternity. I knew that Igor had not been feeling well lately. Everybody thought that he had an allergic reaction to an antibiotic. But I knew right then what he meant. My friend had just been diagnosed with the most aggressive, insidious, mortal type of lymphoma that exists. His cancer had almost a non-existing survival rate in spite of the most advanced chemotherapy available. I wept, hugged and prayed with him for the longest time.

"How long, Igor?"

"Three years top, Mercy. No more. *Statistics don't lie.*

"But there's the power of prayer, we don't know what God has in store for you! Don't give up, please."

"Just pray that I spend purgatory down here baby, just pray for that." He embraced me tightly and left.

Igor's illness added a new perspective to our domestic liaison. We were pressured to make a decision as to acquire his old property or to buy another one. Igor started receiving aggressive chemo treatments weekly. It was the end of 2003. There was an illusion of a seeming reduction of enlarged lymph nodes but it was short-lived. Igor's cancer took a turn for the worst.

By early 2004, to aggravate our situation the national housing market was booming like never before in history. Cheap mortgage rates plus lenders willing to qualify any potential buyers even at the cost of infamous adjustable rate-mortgages fueled the market into a real-estate buying frenzy. The economy was relatively strong, healthy, and unemployment was low; both national and foreign investors got over-confident. Continued home appreciation brought Igor's former house into an astonishing new market value. The house more than doubled its original price. We did not have the funds to purchase Igor's old property. The boom was in full swing and we did not have the monetary resources to comply. The deal was canceled.

We immediately began our desperate search for another place to live. In a downright seller's market where demand was much larger than supply, we faced an almost impossible feat. As prices skyrocketed we knew we could not afford a house; we had to settle for a modest apartment.

Several months passed and every time we thought we were closed to finalize a deal, the apartment we had our eyes set on was snatched right from our fingers by a more aggressive buyer. One afternoon, I received a telephone call from my country. It was from my only uncle on my maternal side alive. The house where I was born and raised in Cuba, the house that my grandfather, a very accomplished architect in Havana, had built with his own company and was full of all the amenities money could buy in the 50's, the house that stored all my childhood memories and most importantly, all of my childhood's true expressions of love from my aunts and uncle and grandmother had been finally sold to a stranger by a considerable amount of dollars.

Although by that time, my grandmother, my two aunts and my loved uncle and godfather who had brought me up had long passed away; the somber news was a reaffirmation that my childhood had been officially buried. Eternally.

I am officially the oldest generation of my family. The sense of loss that overtook me was immense. That house represented the first chapter of my life and it had been finally closed. That same night I went to bed around ten. I was tired and fell fast asleep.

Around three in the morning I suddenly woke up. I let out a screeching sound. My left ear was all clogged up. I felt like I was submerged in a deep sea water tank, far and down from the surface, all reminiscence of sound left on the surface meters away from me. Only I was not in a tank, there was no oxygen equipment, no mask, no swooshing waves, and no bubbles. No sign of water. I was at home, on the ground, on my bed, screaming to the top of my lungs and I could not hear anything on my left side. It was a horrible sensation. My husband and my kids came rushing to my side. "I am deaf. I am deaf! That was all I could shout." I felt no pain, no ringing, no hissing, no nothing, just a strange hollowness inside my head that did not allow me to perceive any sound at all. I was sucked in a deafening silent vacuum.

I cried. I cried out of fear. And then I had to accept that at that time of the night there was nothing else I could do. I had to wait until morning to visit my family doctor. I sobbed and whimpered until weariness led me to an undisturbed sleep.

Around eight in the morning I opened up my eyes and the absolute deafness on my left ear was still there. It was not a dream; it was not a temporary situation. It was vividly present and most of all it was scary. I dressed up as quickly as I could, fetched my kids to school and sped away in our car to see my primary doctor. He examined me and told me that I was suffering from SHL, sudden hearing loss. The cause? It was unknown but most likely it was a herald of my progressing Meniere. I needed to see a neurotologist as soon as I could. If caught on time, intratympanic steroid injections could improve my hearing, in some rare cases even return it to its previous normal range.

I made an emergency appointment to see a famous physician at Baptist Hospital and I was seen the very next day. The doctor was a tall, slim, and gray-haired renowned ear specialist in Florida, Dr. Lawrence Grobman (he is indeed a Neurotologist and my ENT up to present) who discussed at length with me what my primary doc had just explained. Steroid shots in the affected ear could improve my hearing or have no beneficial effect at all, but the sooner it was treated the better chance I had to recover some hearing back.

I took a series of intratympanic steroid shots in my left ear (also called perfusion therapy). By the third treatment, as soon as the topical anesthesia, lidocaine, reached my ear drum and the small needle delivered the dexamethasone-steroid injection I could not control the short-lasting but ferocious vertigo. I hardly made it to the sink in the small office and emptied all my stomach contents in it. I left the office in pain, in tears, and walking assisted by my husband. I swore to myself never to have those shots again.

It did not matter though, if three injections could not reverse the damage to the ear, no greater amount of steroids would do it. For the next few days, vertigo lingered around. I had no much balance either. It was shot but it all subsided in about a week. When I came two weeks later to have my hearing checked on my left ear I had recovered about one third of my hearing ability. The shots had worked after all, at least partially. Ironically, when I started losing my hearing ten years ago, my right ear was the one at fault. Now, in 2004, I had my SHL in my left ear. For the last ten years I had been answering the phone with my left ear. It had all changed in matter of hours. From that day on, if I wanted to speak via a telephone I had to use my right ear. Baffling, ironic, spooky but that's the way it was. In addition, I would have to sit with my "good ear", which of course was hearing impaired as well, near the person I was with if I wanted to understand the words spoken to me And I'd have to become an expert at lip reading, especially if the language in question was English. When you lose hearing as much as I did, you have to face a great challenge for the rest of your life. Losing hearing ability means that for the rest of your life you will struggle to understand the world around you, you will become totally disoriented as to what direction a sound comes from and amazingly, you will be bothered by background noise that everyone else automatically tunes out.

Why sudden deafness strikes, and whom, remains a mystery. Nobody knows. Some clinicians seem to believe that it's all due to a viral infection, others that it is a case of an autoimmune disease (own body attacks hearing system). In my case, it was attributed to my progressing Meniere; an inevitable characteristic of this sinister illness.

The faster SHL is treated with corticosteroids the greater the chance to recover at least some of the hearing lost. The steroids decrease inflammation and may increase labyrinthine circulation. That is the main theory behind its use in both Meniere's severe bouts of vertigo and complete sudden deafness. For obvious reasons, only a well-trained neurotologist is fully accredited to deliver these ear injections.

Whether it was Igor's illness, the pressure to find a new dwelling, the news from Cuba that sharpened my reality as the "oldest generation" or a combination of all of the above, the truth is that my good ear had become ill too. My disease had advanced. Unbeknownst to me, I had changed my status. I had officially become *a bilateral Menierian.* The destructive condition was now present in both my ears.

By the end of year 2004, we purchased and moved into an over-priced three bedroom apartment near my husband's place of work. In January 2005, Igor succumbed to lymphoma. I recovered from my shot balance, the loss of my affectionate friend and adapted to my further hearing deterioration as best as I could. I got fitted with a new digital programmable hearing aid, courtesy of my son's school Key Club group. (Key Club is the oldest and largest service program for high school students and it is a student-led organization whose goal is to teach leadership through service to others.) Key Club's gesture was a great help indeed; most insurance policies do not cover hearing aid purchases. I kept moving on with my life but I could not possibly fathomed what awaited me in a not so distant future as a *Bilateral Menierian, the most challenging, baffling and bedeviled condition an otolaryngologist might encounter during his whole career.*

CHAPTER 22

✦

BACK IN THE SWIRL

Swirl. Vanilla, strawberry swirls, ice-cream. Those are the words that used to flush my mind whenever I thought about the world swirl. Images from my memory lane trip. The craving of a vanilla ice-cream topped with strawberry swirls; the cold refreshing flavor of the frozen sweet snack contrasting the warm glass of water and the sordid heat that enveloped the long streets to be walked day after day to come back and forth from my high school institute in my country.

Vanilla was the most common flavor served in Cuba in those days. All Cubans had grown justly tired of it. We all craved other delicacies. I, personally, would have given anything to have a delicious whole covered strawberry icy dessert in my mouth but next to it the vanilla concoction adorned with swirling streams of the real deal, strawberries, seemed the next best option. They were an exotic luxury in my country like most anything else be it food or clothing or well . . . anything else really covers it all.

Swirl. Alternating shades of fuchsia and magenta and rosy pink

A few years later.
November 4th, 2007 to be exact. My 46th birthday. It should have been a typical day in my ordinary life. At least that's what I thought when I made plans for my celebration day the week before. I went to commemorate it at Eli's house. I wanted to be with her

and her family on that important occasion as we always gathered together to celebrate all major festivities in our lives. I had left my country in 1980. Nine years after my departure, Eli, by then married and with a 3 year old beautiful kid, was able to migrate to this country and established her residence in Miami as well. Our friendship took an interlude of nine years but it was simply a brief pause in our lives. We'd finally reconnected and strengthened the bond that we had been cultivating since we first met in middle school.

Nothing particularly eventful early on that day took place that I can recall but it's safe to assume that an unhealthy stress had been lurking in my life lately. My children were all fast approaching the turbulence of adolescence, my marriage had already started the pathway too often traveled by disintegrating families. Any outsider could have been blinded to the real intimate status of my matrimony. I was the first one to be taken aback by the reality of our relationship's doom but it was there, covered in well-kept appearances but there nonetheless. It was just a matter of time, the proverbial ticking-bomb; one that for sure was about to explode into powerful, devastating thousand pieces destroying everything on its path, especially my children and my own health. And it exploded; eventually it burst and shattered all of our lives. Being that the current state of affairs it was only safe to assume that I was immersed in a ripe, fertile soil for what I was about to experience.

I watched the kids, mine and Elizabeth, jumping around, flipping in the air, splashing everything around as they took a dive into Eli's pool. Most years, November weather in Miami is as hot and pleasant for a refreshing cool dive as in August. I heard the kids' laughter, their sounds of contentment and I sighed with joy.

We, the adults, were seated in the Spanish-tiled covered backyard terrace savoring the lazy Sunday afternoon. I took a sip

163

from my chilled, pink-lemonade beverage. I dragged a puff of my Virginia Slim. Just then, I felt it; the familiar ringing, the buzzing and the strange feeling that overcame me in a split second; the general malaise that preceded the attack that would flip my life around one more time. I could have never fathomed the challenge I was about to encounter . . . all over again.

I dismissed the signs nevertheless and attempted to eat some of the food that was selected for the occasion; Imperial rice, a typical Latin dish of yellow rice cooked with chicken and covered with melted Gouda cheese all over it. I managed to gulp down some of it. A new nausea wave invaded me. I went inside and lied down on Ada's bed (Eli's mom). I summoned my friend to fetch a Xanax from my purse. I popped one in. I tried to close my eyes. Vertigo did not allow it. I waited a while staring at the ceiling COMPLETELY MOTIONLESS, NOT DARING TO SWIVEL MY HEAD ONE INCH OVER TO ANY SIDE OF THE BED. I popped in a second Xanax pill.

My vertigo seemed to abate after a while and I went back to the dining room. Ada served me a slice of a delectable, appetizing, cold strawberry cheesecake, my old-time favorite American dessert. It looked as good as it tasted. It was homemade from scratch with crunchy Graham crackers crumbs on the bottom, strawberry sauce covering the creamy cheesecake and a swirl of whipped cream on top. Everybody clasped their hands together and sang in unison the tunes of the most sung song in the history of the world. In an atmosphere of sheer enthusiasm and camaraderie I took a glance at the cheesecake delicious swirls of alternating shades of magenta and fuchsia. I enjoyed the vision with sheer delight.

As soon as I had finished eating I went back to the terrace and right then, I was caught in the grip of a newer, stronger attack. I did not wait any longer and bolted for our van. I remember yelling to the kids to hurry up and join me. The kids toweled off their slick bodies and changed into their dry clothes. From a distance I heard my husband's grunts. He was fuming, how did I dare to spoil his Sunday break, his day of indulgence, (never mind it was *my entitled day of indulgence too*) with one of my presumptive nonsense episodes? I made an effort and stuck my hand out of the van and waved goodbye at my friends.

The trip back home was a hell of a ride. The attack gained intensity very rapidly. By the time, I reached our parking lot, a good 45 minutes from Eli's house, I was rendered a functioning vegetable. Does such a thing even exist? Squealing and moaning I surrendered myself completely to my kids. Adrian and Mercy Jr. grabbed me under my arms and literally dragged me all the way to our elevator. Once inside, I could not hold it anymore. With the force of a potent projectile out it went my hardly digested Imperial rice and my delicious cheesecake. My daughter Mercy wiped out my lifeless face. I felt sorry for Ben, our building maintenance man. I could imagine his disgusted face when he was summoned to clean my mess by an outraged neighbor. By the time my kids opened up our front door, my disequilibrium was complete and in that state I was launched onto my bed where my sweet baby changed my dirty clothes and brought a bucket to my rescue. For the next ten hours the same painstaking activities were repeated over and over in my bedroom; my cries filling out the whole room. Poor my sweet baby-cake; she was only thirteen at the time but she had always acted more mature than her age; well, "almost always". My baby made sure that whatever anti-anxiety medication I had access to was swallowed hastily in order to put a stop to the horrific scenario.

The Swirls, the strawberry ice-cream grungy swirls from my teenage years danced in my brain, twirling, swaying, taunting me; see Mercy? We are so delicious! Catch us if you dare! The celebratory cheesecake slices' pinkish swirls were added to the burlesque parade in my mind, I heard the strawberry swirls laughter; you like us, don't you Mercy? You like the swirls? Here, have some of your own and they kept on going round and around and some more and I wanted them to stop, I wanted to tell them that I was not enjoying their pretentious spectacle anymore but they kept on their uncoordinated pirouettes reluctant to follow a stop command.

Before the pharmaceuticals overpowered the malevolent swirls and rendered them still I had one last thought.

Mercy, after all of your sickness free-years, all your confidence about being symptom-free, all the reassurance that you have conquered and prevailed you are back to being the poor-disabled-afflicted by relentless vertigo-Mercy.

Mercy, you are back, Back in the swirl of . . . Meniere.

CHAPTER 23

— ❀ —

SURPRISE, SURPRISE

A few days later my vertigo seemed to be a little under control. My son had decided to enroll at a dual program in our community college campus and I was able to accompany him to Open House night. My friend Olga went with us just as a backup for me. I barely made it through the night but I gathered all the required transcripts and paper work needed for his transfer to the new program the next day.

Alas, the good fortune did not last long. For the next few months a horror film was displayed before my eyes. I became both spectator and reluctantly-active-participant at the same time. I re-lived in full color the same agony of sixteen years ago. Attacks gained intensity, strength, and duration with each passing day. It was the same inherent anxiety buildup as the one that we, people who live in country-affected-hurricane areas experience each new season.

It felt just like watching a tropical disturbance forming in the coasts of Africa, watching it slowly gaining intensity, becoming more and more organized, progressing over the torrid Atlantic waters until it metamorphoses into an unstoppable monster of a hurricane with winds of 155 miles per hour or more; a category-five monster, capable to irrefutably destroy everything on its path as soon as it touches land. Unlike a hurricane, however, Meniere crises do not subside in one or two days, no, they can stay for years yes, not one day, week or even a month but years at a time. At least that has been my own, particular painful experience.

Just like many too years ago when Meniere made its first appearance in my life, I missed Misa de Gallo on Christmas Eve of year 2007. My favorite celebration of the year was dampened by a severe crisis. I spent more than 20 hours all curled up in fetal position in my bed, unable to tilt my head a centimeter so not to aggravate the rebellious vertigo. I tried Xanax and Benadryl combined but vomiting was relentless. I am lost at words to explain the horror of being rendered immobile and yet suffering excruciatingly vertigo, knowing that no medication can do a thing for you. Add to the sorrowful spectacle the prying eyes of three young lives who had not a clue as to why their once "normal" mommy was lying in bed, present and absent all the same, sick, unreachable, stolen from them.

The feeling of abandonment, perceived as real although not intentional on my part, was too intense for my kids to sustain and the consequential detrimental effect imposed on my children by my ordeal will reveal itself in years to come.

As New Year rolled over, I decided to seek Hismanal as a continuous and foolproof treatment, and why not? Meniere had come back to stay and Hismanal had proven victorious against it some number of years before. I paid a visit to the local neurotologist that I saw back in 2004 when I had my sudden hearing loss, Dr. Grobman, to request a prescription.

"I am sorry—Dr. Grobman said but Hismanal has been banned by FDA for quite some time now."

My mouth fell open into a sour curl. I was left aghast.
My heart started racing,

"Then, what's going to happen to me? Is there any other drug available to substitute Hismanal?"

"No." My doc said. Astemizole, (the pharmaceutical name for Hismanal), has been withdrawn from USA market due to rare but unfortunate patient cases of cardiac side effects events including death, and severe arrhythmias. However, Betahistine, commercially known as Serc is a widely used medicine in Europe and Canada to treat Meniere's

Dare to give it a try?"
"Of course!"

Although Serc is one of those medicines that are not sold in your everyday pharmacy but only at compound pharmacies I found one relatively close to my home and my husband had it filled out right away.

I started taking Serc at the maximum dose allowed; three times a day. One week passed by, then two, and three and . . . no change. To my dismay, my condition kept worsening by the day. On top of my constant malaise, I started suffering from GERC (gastroesophageal reflux disease) simply known as acid reflux; a condition in which backward flow of acid from the stomach causes heartburn and damage to the esophagus, the tube that connects the mouth to the stomach. It was a side effect of so many medications taken in a lying position and so much vomiting damaging my esophagus lining. The constant burning sensation added more misery to my already battered body. Tums and Pepcid tablets were then added to my daily medicinal regimen.

My life turned into an inferno. How much longer I have to endure these implacable, atrocious, demoniac attacks Lord? I queried every day. But I had no answer, just absolute, painful silence, as days turned into nights and nights into days. I was either sound asleep from all my meds or vomiting and caught up in a constant head *swirling*, mastering the art of *trying to sleep through it all*. The vicious attacks rendered me in a semi-comatose, sort of a zombie-breathing soul with no quality of life left in my disease-savaged body. Everything in my life had been ripped out from under me once again and whether I realized it or not I had begun another journey of unmitigated hell.

CHAPTER 24

—— ✺ ——

YEAR 2008

As my condition further deteriorated, I was rushed in an ambulance to the nearest ER on several occasions in the month of March. My days and nights were spent lying down in bed doing absolutely nothing but watching my bedroom's ceiling move in circles and vomiting continuously. I simply could not lie on my left side, the severe vertigo episodes will not allow it; I was forced to lie on my right side for twenty hours at a stretch. It was nearly impossible to sleep or rest, my muscles were all tied up in knots exhausted from trying to combat and arrest the never ending circular motion that engulfed me at all times. Whatever sleep I had is was all forced on me from medicine side effects and it was just not enough to restore my ill body.

In a flannel gown and in a wheelchair with my limp head hanging to a side (impossible to keep it straight when seized by an attack) I was wheeled into my ENT office. He prescribed Zofran (Ondansetron) for nausea, Valium for vertigo attacks, Phenergan suppositories for the vomiting and of course, Dyazide to help out with fluid retention.

The meds helped a little bit to control attacks but either way, I was condemned to live in my bed as an invalid. Like in the 80s, just trying to get in and out of bed required a titanic effort, nausea always worsened when I moved my head. Going to the loo was an "impossible mission." I dreaded every time I had to go. I knew I would end up throwing up no matter how carefully I moved.

Eli, my dear friend, came to my rescue. She bought me a portable commode and placed it right by my bed. We baptized the new chair as "the throne." Now, the trip to the oval chair had been shortened and consequently, the vomiting frequency. I learned by trial and error to wait for my meds to kick in to lift up myself out of bed very carefully and make it to the "royal chair."

Eli also provided me with other lifesaving objects such as an under mattress foam wedge to help raise my bed, sturdy grab bars with super strong PVC suctions cups to attach to bathroom tiles and/or walls (can't tell you how many times I was seized by a spell while showering and instinctively I reached out for the curtain shower to hold on to it to avoid falling down, genius right?), a long reach plastic stick that I used to wipe myself in places I couldn't reach when the slightest movement on my part triggered an intense nausea wave and finally, a bath bench to avoid any accidents while in the tub. As a bonus she shopped for a new stove for me and had her dear hubby installed it. My old kitchen range had a broken oven; and a totally functioning stove is an invaluable asset when you suffer from Meniere, has 3 young kids to feed and need to fix simple dinners amidst relentless spinning vertigo! God bless Eli! If only I would have had all those useful assisting living items when Meniere first appeared in my youth!

My late mother-in-law who passed away in 1999, had left behind a walker. I placed it within reach and never ventured anywhere without it. Since I was literally living in my bed, my nightstand became my desk-medicine cabinet-tray table and telephone station all in one. I kept all my meds, cell phone, charger, snacks, water, juices, laptop and pen and paper readily accessible on top of my nightstand. I became an expert at stretching out my hand and reaching for the needed object at a particular time. My sense of touch guided me since I could not swivel my head to look for any desired object. Right by my bedside, I kept a plastic bucket, clean towels, a box of wipes and some lavender eau de cologne, much needed articles when vomiting is part of your daily routine!

Those early months of year 2008 were very hard on my children but this was also a time when there was an outpour of abundant blessings over our household. I, for once, received a one-sided VIP treatment from parents from both my daughters' school and from my Emmaus' prayer group. (My Emmaus prayer group is comprised of mothers from the school my son attended in his junior high years.)

Moms and dads equally, okay more moms than dads took turns to bring us a hot meal every single day of the week. They even coordinated a schedule that worked magnificently. Every morning I received a call to inform me of the family who will cater to us and the "menu" for the day. Did my kids eat pasta? Veggies? Any allergies? The parents were so kind, compassionate and thoughtful that I will never forget their generous gesture. It was a huge relief for my children and I to have supper every day while I was severely incapacitated.

Olga was by my side faithfully. Many too a day she came home to sweep the floor, clean the bathrooms, cook some dinners to be stored for the weekends when help from school took a break and to take Mercy Jr. to the market to do some light grocery shopping. Many of my prayer group friends came over to visit me, to pray with me, to bring me flowers, to cheer me up and to let me know they cared about me; all gestures that were deeply appreciated and that brought me a lot of comfort.

Meanwhile, I kept searching for answers and new treatments. Since Hismanal is an anti-histaminic and it had worked wonders for me in the past I gave it a try at some OTC anti-histamines. I tried Benadryl, Allegra and Zyrtec at different intervals. None of them, unfortunately, rose to the challenge.

Benadryl, being the oldest soldier in the company and the cheapest one seemed to alleviate my symptoms just a little bit but it was a far cry from the relief I was seeking. Allegra did not do anything for me and Zyrtec just induced a very strange side effect on me. It lowered my blood pressure to very unstable values. By the third time my BP went down to 60/40 I gave up on it entirely.

I extended my search to the much obliged enlightenment of a second medical opinion. I directed my steps, no matter how wobbly they were, to the University of Miami Otology Department, talk about reliving an experience! Dr. Andrell, the ENT assigned to my case, ordered a vast comprehensive but fastidious balance tests and a new audiometry.

The tests were tedious, extremely uncomfortable and worst of all designed to provoke vertigo on purpose to determine the extension of the inner ear damage. Imagine, what this ordeal means to a patient who lives in a rotational spinning circle everyday of her life!

To add salt to the wound, I had to stop taking all anti-vertigo medications three days prior to testing day to ensure the most accurate results possible. Talk about an insurmountable feat. I knew right off the bat I could not do it on my own. I turned to my prayer group for intercession and they had my back. Ah, the power of prayer!

All in all, it took me around two months to complete all testing. I survived them all without vomiting. I only experienced a minor dizziness that resolved promptly. The tests did not reveal anything new. Both my ears were severely affected by Meniere. The UM doc did not have a new treatment for me but miraculously by the time I was done with all the exams it was already summer and Meniere bid me farewell of its own accord. Just like that.

I felt giddy, intoxicated with sheer joy and took advantage of my regained "illness-free status". I went about restoring my body strength and enjoying life with great enthusiasm. I swam in my building pool until well advanced in the night hours. I visited the gym religiously. I cooked, I shopped, I went to restaurants but my lucky break was interrupted by an emergency microsurgery to remove a lumbar herniated disc.

Summer season ended, school routine settled in and by September I was recuperated enough to face the world again. On September 24th, 2008, I attended a very interesting Philosophical Forum at my school's son. All of my friends complimented me on how great I looked.

Did they jinx it for me? Of course, I am kidding but by the very next day I was back in the treacherous web of Meniere's vertigo. In the ensuing months, the attacks became as vicious as before. Year 2009 ended in the same grimly way it commenced.

CHAPTER 25

— ✦ —

YEAR 2008, STEPPING UP THE GAME

As soon as the New Year began, I knew I had to take a painful but not entirely novel step in my life. I enlisted my ENT's help and entered a new application to receive a disabled status by the Florida Social Security Administration. This time around, there was no need for appeals, hearings or anything of the sort. When I received the letter acknowledging my new disabled granted status, I didn't know exactly if it was a curse or a blessing but it was clear that my precarious health was nothing to be taken lightly. The swift answer from SSA confirmed it. Go ahead, ask around and see how many people can claim a disabled status from SSA just the very first time they apply for it. Remember how it took me almost three years back in the 80s to finally get it? So, hats off to my clinician and his staff for supplying all the required medical documentation to the pertinent authorities. No hats off to Meniere though. The villain did not deserve it.

A word of advice to all Menierians and/or chronic ill readers out there; do not attempt to apply for disability benefits unless you are firmly backed up by records from a registered, Board certified, medical practitioner or preferably a specialist with years of expertise in your condition. The more diagnostics tests and scans you can provide to substantiate your case, the better for your claim. In the specific example of Meniere I highly recommend a letter from either an Otolarygonlogist or better yet, a Neurotologist.

Although I expected to be enrolled in the Medicare program as soon as I was declared incapacitated it was not meant to be so. By Florida law, I learned I had to wait until January 2011, two years later, to automatically be enrolled in Medicare. Oops, my mistake! Actually, I had to wait twenty four consecutive months "after" I started to receive benefits to be enrolled in the Medicare program, totaling the amount of months without medical insurance to a good thirty months. (I was declared disabled in January 2009. I did not begin to receive any benefits until six months later.) That was correct. I had to wait until July 2011 to be a Medicare recipient. The only exceptions in the Sunshine state are those patients with renal failure. In those cases, Medicare coverage starts immediately.

My heart goes out to all disabled people who need medical attention because of diverse serious health conditions, are unable to work and therefore do not have medical insurance through a workplace and on top of their misfortune they have no medical coverage at all for two or three or whatever amount of years they have to wait! I was fortunate at the time I applied for disability to be covered through my husband's employer medical insurance program but eventually my marriage of almost 20 years disintegrated and I lost all coverage. (We can't trust men with anything really important!) In the end, my divorce was postponed on account of this highly inconvenient obstacle and I ended up refunding my ex for my own medical premium until Medicare kicked in. Did I mention how unreliable men are? Yes, I did. No further comments.

On a much happier note, the parent's network from my daughters' school kept a steadfast support. A certain mom eagerly volunteered to chauffeur me to a holistic practice and pay for the first visit services. As much as I desired to try on anything new, I had to decline the generous offer. I was too ill to brave the frequent trips to a holistic practitioner on a regular basis. A holistic approach requires as much commitment as going to psychotherapy if you want to reap some fruits. I was severely incapacitated. Financially speaking, it was not feasible either. I passed on the opportunity. Nevertheless, if you are in the position to afford an alternative medical treatment I think you will have nothing to lose and plenty to gain.

Procedures and methods such as acupuncture, homeopathic treatments and soothing massages may relieve some of your symptoms and improve your overall sense of well-being. Meniere, by its intrinsic nature, robs its victims of all sense of control over their lives. By being proactive in your recovery, not only you will attain a better quality of life but will regain some of that lost control too.

A fair advice, do some serious research about the professional you plan to visit. If he's highly recommended by a friend or relative so much the better!

Another mom connected me with a lady who had suffered from Meniere for many moons like me. Her name was Lisa Anderson. Lisa and I exchanged tons of Meniere information over the web in the following months. Lisa is the only bilateral Menierian that I have met personally. Like me, she had battled this monster for decades. Her symptoms were not as severe as mine but when seized by an attack she would be bedridden for weeks also.

Lisa suggested me to step up my game and I paid heed to her advice. I went back to see my ENT and asked him for a new approach to treat my Meniere. I was placed on an oral steroid treatment for several weeks. To my dismay, the steroids only made me gain weight and that was all I got out of the whole thing; talk about being proactive!

Refusing to be disheartened I advanced one more step; a new round of steroid shots in my left ear, the one that lost all hearing ability back in 2004 remember? This time around I was not the "new kid in town." I knew exactly what to expect so . . . I armed myself with anti-nausea meds prior to the procedure and I just experienced a minor and brief discomfort. Yay! I survived the shots but my joy was short-lived. I was dizzy-free for two entire . . . . days after my second shot and that was the end of it.

I want all my readers to bear in mind that many Menierians benefit from these steroid treatments and their vertigo subside considerably after they receive the injections. But as I have mentioned before, Meniere is a very capricious disease; it's tricky, devilish and not two single people react the same to treatments not do they experience all symptoms with the same severity.

Unwilling to be discouraged, I turned my search for a cure to other venues. My next inquiry was in the field of research or experimental clinical trials for Meniere. With the help of this century database guru, the internet, I found out about several ongoing Meniere trials. One of them seemed to hit the target. It was intended for bilateral Menierians. It aimed to control otherwise unabated and continuous vertigo. I contacted Pfizer at once (the pharmaceutical company sponsoring the trial) via e-mail. Although I seemed to qualify for the trial, much to my chagrin, it turned out to be an impossible love, sort of a Romeo and Juliet affair; the trial was being conducted in Australia. Enough said. Shattered dreams.

Sildenafil, the drug being tested by Pfizer in this particular study, resounded in my ears like a very familiar chemical compound. Lo and behold, when I further researched the drug, its commercial name turned out to be none other than Viagra! Surprise, surprise! What do ears have in common with . . . Well, your guess is as good as mine!

Undeterred in my quest (more like desperate I admit), I applied the old adage . . . "If the mountain does not come to me . . . . Let **me** come to the mountain" or something like that. Remember, English is just my second language. What I am about to recount, I DO NOT RECOMMEND IT FOR YOU TO DO AT HOME. I REPEAT LIKE TV STUNT'S COMMERCIALS, "DON'T TRY THIS AT HOME"

Fair warning. Yes you have guessed by now what I did. Being the conservative lady I am, I decided to snatch a couple of Viagra's pills laying around the house and give it a go but not at full dosage. I warned my two oldest children before they left for school about my experiment as an extra precautionary measure and as soon as they marched out of the house I downed half one of those "miraculous pills of new modern medicine". About a good half an hour later my cheeks got red as a fire truck and I also felt a steam coming up my neck, especially around my ears. They both were all as red as cherry tomatoes and my face burned as if engulfed by a fire that needed to be put out by the aforementioned fire truck. To my further detriment, my heart started galloping so fast that if it would have been a favorite solid-hoofed-domesticated-herbivorous-quadruped-stallion aka, horse, at the Kentucky derby; it could have won first prize undoubtedly. *Lady, you need to slow down or this thing is going to do you for good I warned myself.*

I lied down in my bed and waited for my unexpected symptoms to subside. Kids will always be, well . . . kids. As soon as mine rushed back from school they asked me at unison all the while grinning wide.

"How did it go mom?"

"Oh, not as well as I expected it but . . . . I am keeping my hopes high" And that's exactly what I did. The very next day I, an audacious soldier, cut up half a pill into another half and down it with some water. Intrepid soldiers never lose hope! Fifteen minutes elapsed and no dangerous symptoms, hooray! But fifteen more later . . . I had the same worrisome reactions as before. Soldier defeated. I surrendered my arms to the enemy, (Meniere).

It is my most deep desire that scientists may strike a winner in Viagra and that many Menierians if not all may benefit completely from its anti-vertigo properties in case this is just a solid achievement in the anti-Meniere noble cause. I might even adventure to say that if proven a solid relief Viagra would make many male Menierians and their partners as well extremely content; they might kill two birds with the same stone you might say. Nonetheless, this is clearly a path I had to steer away from; the short-time side effects proved to be unbearable in my case. There's only one thing left to say here. This foray into the unexplored territory of clinical trials just earned me a new nickname, Dumbo. That's right, my children baptized me after the famous Disney pachyderm. I don't think I need to explain myself any further!!!!

CHAPTER 26

❧

YEAR 2009, SARASOTA AND THE SILVERSTEIN INSTITUTE

S pring break 2009 was fast approaching and I was still constantly spinning; no respite in sight. As luck would have it, yet another mother from my girls' school (yes, I know I sound like a magician pulling bunnies out of his hat, the way I keep bringing different mothers from my daughters' school into this story). Well, this particular mom's father happened to be a long time Meniere veteran too. For many years, he suffered horrendously from the devilish accompanying vertigo until the day he visited the Silverstein Institute and the Ear Research Foundation in Sarasota, Florida. There, Dr. Herbert Silverstein, the founder and director, performed a surgery in his affected ear that cured him completely of his vertigo.

Dr. Silverstein, an international renowned Otologist, has been constantly recognized since 1979 as one of "The Best Physicians in the USA". He has been a leader in Otology for more than 25 years, developing surgical and diagnostic procedures such as the Microwick system and the facial nerve monitor stimulator. He had also taught a myriad of colleagues, residents and medical students helping people from all walks of life. He is internationally regarded as a leading authority on Meniere's disease. It will take me many pages to name all of his career achievements. Suffice it to say that in 1979, he founded the Silverstein Institute where he serves as a both a physician/ mentor and a researcher. In addition, he is also a celebrated jazz musician and proceeds from his albums and concerts are entirely donated to advance research at his Institute.

I received his information as a sign from heaven. I wasted no time. I submitted all my medical records and tests, yes, quite a few pages as you can imagine, and booked an appointment with Dr. Silverstein that coincided with my daughters' school Spring break. Since my Meniere was present in both ears I knew I was not a candidate for surgery. My heart was set though in Dr. Silverstein's minimally invasive Microwick procedure, a technique that allows patients to treat themselves at home with minimum discomfort. The Wick, implanted at the doctor's office, absorbs the medication and delivers it to the inner ear. Patients may administer medications via drops up to three times a day.

I, enthusiastically, expected to have one of those Wicks implanted in my left ear and had it treat it with gentamicin, an antibiotic that deaden the inner ear in severe cases of vertigo that do not respond to more conventional treatments (in plain English, myself).

It's considered a last resort treatment but with less side effects than surgery and yes, they are effective in stopping vertigo in the 90th percentile range. The downside? Gentamicin might further destroy residual hearing and of course, balance might be affected too. Well, after two years of continuous, unabated vertigo "gentamicin" sounded like a genuine option and perhaps the only one available to me.

Dr. Silverstein ordered all the extensive and expected routine tests. Due to lack of funds and time (on my part, of course,) allergy tests were not provided.

Dr. Silverstein firmly believes that in many Meniere cases there is an allergic component that needs to be addressed as well. Is that why Hismanal, an anti-histaminic, worked wonders for me back in the 80s? I wish I knew with certainty.

When all results were back in the good doctor's hands, he pronounced the words I did not want to hear. I was not a candidate for the gentamicin treatment. My left ear had almost no hearing left; the right one had its balance system mostly destroyed. Dr. Silverstein would not dare to proceed with gentamicin. In his own words, and I quote him "You could end up walking like a duck and you wouldn't be happy with me, would you?"

Bilateral Meniere had left me with no good ear to take over the destroyed balance in the treated ear. In other words, I would be like a person with just one functional kidney that decides to donate it as any Good Samaritan will do. But would this Good Samaritan have a spare good kidney to take over the body cleaning process that BOTH kidneys are in charge of? Of course not. Neither did I have a good ear. No Biblical story for me.

I felt as a helium balloon that after proudly parades around a kid's much awaited birthday's festivities; then, it's suddenly caught up in the grips of a pair of scissors carelessly lying around and Oops! Down comes balloon from its ethereal glory. The kid cries his eyes out. The balloon is totally deflated. So was I.

With nothing further to add, I bid Dr. Silverstein farewell. I clutched my walker firmly, my girls held my handbag. We stopped to reimburse the good doc for his professional services on the way out. I was handed out my prescriptions. His fees were pretty decent taking into consideration all the tests he ordered and his consultation time. God bless him. It was the third time I had encountered such a compassionate soul in the medical field in all of my years battling Meniere.

I was prescribed Ativan, which is similar to Valium but dissolves under your tongue working faster in case of an acute attack, and a recommendation to see a rheumatologist here in Miami. The rheumatologist was instructed to prescribe me Methotrexate pills. I had to be under his constant supervision. Why did I need to see a rheumatologist? Why Dr. Silverstein himself or my old reliable, local ENT could not prescribe methotrexate for me?

Methotrexate or MTX as I would refer to it from now on is a very powerful medicine with potentially serious even fatal adverse side effects. MTX is primarily used to treat autoimmune diseases such as RA (Rheumatoid Arthritis, psoriasis, lupus and others). In much higher doses it is also used in the fight against certain type of cancers.

Dr. Silverstein holds the opinion that bilateral Meniere is an autoimmune condition referred to as AIED (Auto Immune Inner Ear Disease). If Meniere itself is a hardly known ailment among the medical community, AIED is much less so understood and studied. The precise incidence of AIED is highly controversial. It is estimated that as many as 16% of people with bilateral Meniere's disease may suffer from AIED. AIED progressively and consistently destroys hearing function. The patient's own immune system attacks the ear cells recognizing them as "strangers" or "foreigner enemies that need to be put away". How could that be possible? What was wrong with my immune cells anyway? How did my own defense system dare to turn against my own, poor innocent ears instead of external, alien, true gangsters such as bacteria and viruses? Did my immune system go nuts? Well, nobody seems to have the right answer but it appears so, not only in my case but in all auto-immune diseases.

Mostly in meditative and recollected silence I made the trip back home from Sarasota and scheduled an appointment with a local renowned rheumatologist. Following Dr. Silverstein's instructions I was started on a weekly low dosage of MTX and had a baseline lung x-rays and blood tests done.

MTX may cause liver and lung damage among other numerous side effects, therefore, the need to be continuously monitored by a specialist to ensure that you are responding well to treatment and everything is fine. Thanks heaven above I only had a minor initial rash the very first days I took MTX. It pretty soon went away. That was the only secondary reaction I had to MTX. Since MTX weakens the activity of the immune system, as a result, you are more susceptible to catch several infections. If you come down with the flu or any other infection you need to halt treatment until infection is cleared up. I was well informed about all these facts. All it was left for me to do was take the medication as prescribed and wait . . .

As it usually happens with anti-depression treatments, immunosuppressants such as MTX, take a long time to show its effective side and when I say a long time you better believe it is a long time! Although my plans for the Microwick procedure did not materialize, I gave the MTX a fair opportunity to prove its effectiveness. After all, what other choice did I have? Spring Break was over and school resumed.

My status remained about the same for the next 3 months. I spent most days secluded as home as if I were a cloistered nun minus the habit. My secular habit consisted of jammies and slippers mostly.

By the time summer rolled around, I finally caught up a huge break. My ears were not subjected to the constant fullness and pressure as before. The ever present-extremely-annoying-sensation of having "a little man" inside my head pushing it from side to side making me dizzy all the time had become less and less frequent. My disequilibrium was less noticeable too; my energy level went up. In general, the ever present malaise feeling was lifted up like a storm that finally dissipates. My "estranged husband", (my vomiting and vertigo) were finally tamed.

I blessed Dr. Silverstein and all angels around me looking after my well-being. It was time to enjoy the outdoors again.

Summer rays were beaming high in the sky as I plunged into the pool. Sweat dripped down my body as I started bicycling as fast as my body allowed it at the gym. I drove around the neighborhood just to enjoy the view that for so long had evaded me. I met the hustling and bustling of the streets with sheer joy. Nothing like a chronic illness to teach you appreciation for dear life.

In spite of all the fun I was having, three months into MTX treatment I had a relapse. It coincided with the commencement of a new school year. Alarmed, I e-mailed Dr. Silverstein and I poured out my worry unto him. The experienced scientist replied:

"Don't despair. Be consistent. It takes time."

MTX certainly took its sweet time; anywhere from between three to six months before full beneficial effects were experienced. I armed myself with a staunched patience. The rest of the year 2009 marked a new era since the comeback of my fierce opponent. I was still an amazing, intricate, fragile and vulnerable work in progress.

CHAPTER 27

❀

YEAR 2010 UP TO PRESENT . . .

This is my colophon. It has taken me a long time to fill up all of these pages. It has been a laborious project; one of the main anchors that had sustained me throughout my most recent Meniere ordeal. It had also helped me to stifle my legitimate boredom. Along with the most obvious symptoms, Meniere induces an almost chronic fatigue that situates you at either your bed or your couch in the best of instances. A heavy blanket of meds to counteract the vertigo and vomiting reduces you to a zombie-like state.

Reading, watching TV, listening to music (who wants to tune to her I-Pod when ears are ringing, and buzzing like a bee-hive?) and surfing the web for leisure are all activities off-limits. The result? Abrasive boredom; on top of your malaise feeling.

It is then, imperative, to become pro-active in both your treatment and recovery (press hard and push yourself to do any activity when you feel even the smallest improvement) and be highly creative about entertaining yourself and keeping your brain busy.

Writing these pages has been a priceless outlet to my restlessness and my creative juices. Most importantly, it has been an avenue to share my insight and hard-learned lessons about Meniere and clinical depression with all of you. I stated in the previous chapter that at the end of year 2009, I was still a work in progress. I think I will be forever; but I am living a more interesting, satisfying and useful life than in previous years.

I feel like I have tamed and overcome both Meniere and Depression conditions. I feel like a conqueror, victorious, elated, and positively proud of myself.

Year 2009 ended up better than I have envisioned it; yet they were still some hurdles to overcome on my path. A new Caroling season embraced humanity with its splendor. I attended to all the festivities in the company of the family I had created and nurtured for almost twenty years for the last time in my life.

Year 2010 greeted me with severe emotional hardships; the most harrowing one was the final dissolution of my marriage. It won't favor anybody at this junction to recount all the horrors I lived during this period of my life. Perhaps it will be the subject of a new book but for now I will keep the details to myself. None of my children escaped emotionally unscathed from this experience. My divorce was a real prize fight. I felt really terrible for dragging them through all that muck; yet it was completely unavoidable.

By the mid of July 2010, after ten grueling hours spent at the offices of a "Mediator" Family Law attorney my freedom was granted. I was on my own, disabled, penniless and heartbroken all over again. I had two minor children who still needed me although they could have sworn I was totally useless to them. Blame the omniscient teen years. Adolescents view their parents as some sort of "Whatever-Saurus" species who don't know or understand anything about their lives. We are not cool enough; perhaps all parents of pubescent kids should turn into cucumbers to see if they accept us better. Either way, I knew I had to carry on with my life for their sake.

Comprehensibly, all the turmoil I was subjected to during my divorce, kept me in and out of constant Meniere's attacks. I assured you that a great majority of families succumb to the pressures of chronic illnesses, especially one as vicious as Meniere's, but honest to truth my marriage had failed long before Meniere's resurrection.

The day after my marriage was officially dissolved, my symptoms diminish considerably. Change cuts you to the core of your inner being. I think I handled mine pretty well under the circumstances. I moved out of my apartment, rented a new one, furnished it, ran all sorts of errands and filled out all paperwork pertaining to the establishment of new living quarters. I did it all by myself! In all fairness, Olga and Eli lent me their four hands and feet. Mercy Jr.'s role was pivotal. Susan helped . . . at times too. All of my children offered me an incredible support and an unwavering love in spite of their young ages. Eli's husband proved his salt's worth again but it was basically us, women, who did the moving. Pure estrogen power!

When the new school year rolled around, I was able to drive nine miles every afternoon to pick up my girls at their school for the first time in years. It felt awesome.

I could not believe it but immunosuppressants and a more relaxed lifestyle had transformed my life little by little. Ever since then, until present, I have been able to move on and forward at a much easier pace. My days tied down to my bed had diminished considerably. Sitting on my couch in front of a TV set, have become an almost daily part of my life once again. It's great to be in a more erectus position than lying down. It sorts of remind me that I belong to the Homo sapiens species.

I am finally seeing a therapist on a regular basis (welcome CBT, at last!) I am also attending to my prayer group's meetings more frequently. I have been back to the cinema, shopping centers, restaurants and church; all sort of activities and venues that were out of reach for so long. Who knows, there might even be a new guy in my future; a brave soul who wouldn't mind to be my companion in spite of my Meniere's!

As of end of year 2011, I am off MTX. My vertigo is still much more manageable than before.

Now, I do not wish to mislead my readers. I still suffer from Meniere. It has no cure. My disease has steadily progressed throughout the years. My hearing loss is more prevalent and morbid than ever. That is why I am currently fitted with hearing aids in both of my ears. It is really sad, especially not being able to hear my kid's voices like I used to. It is hard when they get frustrated because they have to repeat themselves gazillion times before I can make sense of their uttered words. It is deceitfully dangerous as the time when I went to Ruth Chris Steakhouse restaurant and did not get "Don't touch your steak plate Ma'am; it's very hot!" Ouch! Those are negative consequences. On the plus side, however, a hearing impaired person at the touch of a miniscule button, can't tune out nagging husbands, impatient kids, rebellious teens, whining pets, grouchy bosses, well, you get the picture. Awesome! I don't tend to delve in the loss of my hearing sense. Instead I delight myself in my winnings.

Just being vertigo-free for long periods of times is enough to keep me looking like a smiley-face sticker; brimming a smile from ear to ear. Undoubtedly, when vertigo and dizziness are not present my depression seems to evaporate and my neurons are actively planning all the things I want to do with the rest of my life. All in all, my depression responds very well to treatment. My greatest disability has always been Meniere's not depression, although this scenario might be totally different for both Meniere and Depression patients. Each person is unique and several degrees of these illnesses can manifest in different people.

Oh yes, there are still days when I feel woozy, unbalanced, very weak, my ears ringing and buzzing, fullness and pressure in them and unfortunately dizzy. On those days, I followed the pointers that I have shared with you in this book. I get plenty of rest, take all my meds, cast out all WORRIES, put away my "to do list", meditate, pray and concentrate on my recovery. I know that after raining puppies and kitties, the sun will shine again.

There is one more issue I would like to discuss with all of my females Menierians and their male partners too. This important piece of advice is what I call M&M. No, not the famous-colored mini-chocolates. Unfortunately, it is the intrinsic-Machiavellian relationship between Meniere and Menopause.

If you are a female who suffers from Meniere and you are going through "The Change" you have all my commiseration and admiration. Add an extra portion if you are bilateral like I am. If you are a male who suffer from Meniere thanks all the stars above. You've dodged a good one here.

The Change, Menopause, or better stated yet Perimenopause, (the years before menstruation ceases completely) is certainly a challenging period in most women's lives. It might last between seven to eleven years before you reach actual Menopause. In the case of female Menierians "The Change" might be simply brutal.

Aside from SEVERE MIGRAINE HEADACHES, hot flashes that make us want to strip naked in the middle of the street, night sweats that drench our new 500-thread Ralph Lauren sheets (or the ones we bought at Wal-Mart on sale) prompting us to change them at 3:00 o'clock in the morning followed sometimes by chills that even electric blankets can get rid of, unexpected mood swings, excessive tiredness, hair thinning, irregular cycles that might shorten or lengthen capriciously throwing off our monthly charts, and some other real unpleasant symptoms, we female Menierians have to add one more item to the list: the intensification of our vertigo during this period of our lives.

I am well into my late forties. I have been treading my steps through the rocky ride of Perimenopause for quite a while. I have kept a record of my worst symptoms on a calendar since Meniere came back. I could not help but notice that 95% of the time I suffer from severe symptoms it is always related to my menstrual cycle phases, whether it would be mid-cycle (ovulation), the onset of my period, or the few days prior to it and any other times when I have irregular bleedings. It can't be a coincidence, especially since it is been more noticeable in the last year when MTX has been doing a great job controlling my Meniere!

Younger Menierian females may identify a similar relationship between their cycles and the worsening of their Meniere's symptoms. I am not a doctor but one possible explanation might be the fact that we retain a lot of fluid during some days of our cycles. Most of us get "bloated" prior to our periods onset. Meniere by definition is excess of endolymphatic fluid in the inner ear. Therefore, it should not be surprising that all the water and fluid retention caused by female hormonal fluctuations in our cycles (greatly intensified during Perimenopause) wreak havoc on Meniere female patients.

Could it be possible then, that once that Climacteric (Menopause) finally arrive my Meniere's attacks would considerably decrease in both frequency and duration? I certainly hope so.

In the meantime, I open an extended invitation to the international medical community to join forces, close ranks and come up with groundbreaking answers to both the etiology and cure of Meniere's along with one hundred percent effective treatments to eradicate vertigo.

In the case of female Meniere's patients, clinical researchers should take into account that women are physiologically different from men and that difference affects us significantly in the way we respond to this disease.

Great New News! As I approach the end of this book, Dr. Jay Rubinstein, a surgeon and a biomedical engineer from the University of Washington, has performed an innovative surgery on a male patient who suffers from severe Meniere's recurrent vertigo attacks.

Dr. Rubinstein in cooperation with colleague Dr. James Phillips developed a new device, a vestibular prosthesis that is very similar to a cochlear implant (a device used to help deaf people to hear). With the new modification to the device, the team expects to put a halt to vertigo. Rubinstein's theory is that the vestibular device will supply bursts of electricity to the vestibular nerve to make up for temporarily disabled ear cells. The device should bring perceived spinning by the brain to a stop. A patient should be able to monitor his attacks and bringing to end as soon as they start by manipulating the device in a similar fashion as patients manipulate cochlear implants.

The surgery was the first one of an approved FDA ten-person-clinical trial for the new vestibular apparatus. At present, it has been confirmed that the device stops vertigo in animals. We have to wait and see what it is capable of to do for humans. It is a promisingly and most welcomed news, especially because the procedure does not destroy neither hearing nor balance as more traditional surgeries do. This new procedure, however, is not intended for bipolar Menierians. For more information regarding this clinical trial check the R&R section of this book.

Meniere is a non-terminal illness. The **word *terminal*** has its roots in the Latin word *terminus* which literally means "an endpoint, a place where something ends, a final destination."

Meniere, by definition, it is NOT the end or the final destination of our lives, though it may appear so. It is an affliction that should and can be taken care of. The beauty of Medicine is that is a continuous evolving science; it is always expanding its horizons, it is always giving HOPE.

We have seen an overwhelming outpour of new promising medications being offered to those afflicted by depression in the last few years. An amazing and most welcomed contribution that it was simply unavailable about fifty years ago. I sincerely hope and envision that the same professionalism, dedication and compassion will be displayed by pharmaceutical companies and researchers worldwide to come up with newer and better Meniere treatments and eventually a definite cure. We can't afford to be complacent about the current treatments. There are still many lives that need to be touched by more efficacious and unprecedented treatments.

If I have to summon up my innermost desire for all of you my fellow Menierians, depression sufferers, and all chronically ill people it would be encased in just one word, HOPE.

Never abandon Hope.
Hope for recovery.
Hope for a healthy, vibrant and amazing life.
Amid tragedy, look at your condition as a galvanizing force that offers you the possibility to turn your life around.

It is possible.

"Hope is a thing with feathers
That perches on the soul;
And sings the tune without words
And never stops at all."

Emily Dickinson.

APPENDIX

LATEST NEWS FOR MENIERE.

MR. DANA WHITE, UFC PRESIDENT, HAS REPORTED THAT HE RECEIVED A NEW STEM CELL TREATMENT FOR MENIERE IN GERMANY IN APRIL 2013.

IN HIS OWN WORDS, HE IS 100% CURED.

WE WILL MONITOR MR. WHITE'S RECOVERY VERY CLOSELY

R & R: Recap and Resources

Current, Most Widely Used Meniere Treatments in USA

For acute attacks

Sedatives
Valium (Diazepam), Xanax (Alprazolam), Ativan (sublingual, Lorezipam),

Other anti-vertigo, anti-nausea, anti-emetic (anti-vomiting) medications
Antivert/meclizine
Scopolamine
Zofran/ Ondansetron HCL
Phenergan/ Promethazine (available as pills and suppossitories)

Dramamine/Vomex
Stemetil/Compazine
Vistaril/ Hydroxizine pamoate

Long-term treatment

Diuretics
Dyazide/Maxzide/Maxzide-25
Lasix/Diamox

Doctor might order potassium pills and a diet rich in bananas, oranges, cantaloupes, spinach and sweet potatoes to supplement loss of potassium

Long-term treatment
Serc/ betahistine pills (available at compounding pharmacies)

Dietary manipulation
Low salt (low sodium) diet
Caffeine, alcohol and chocolate restriction

Anti-histamines (after allergy screening is performed)
Allegra
Claritin

Nutritional supplements
Ginko biloba
Lipoflavinoids
Ginger
Second line of treatments/ non-surgical for severe vertigo

Steroids (used both orally and/or intratympanic injections)
Dexamethasone
Prednisone

Second-line/ surgical
Endolymphatic shunt surgery
Endolymphatic sac decompression
Labyrinthectomy

Third-line of treatment for intractable vertigo, non-surgical/ last resort for severe cases of Meniere's

Intratympanic Gentamicin injections
Low-dose and High-dose protocols
Low-dose is most favored protocol as to prevent further hearing loss

Immune suppressants rarely used. They are indicated for AIED syndrome, bilateral Meniere (read chapter 26)

Metothrexate (MTX)
Enbrel

Surgical procedures

Vestibular nerve section
Labyrinthectomy

The Best of the Best/
Renowned physicians and facilities for Meniere's treatment

Current Clinical trial/ Vestibular prosthesis
Dr. Jay Rubinstein/ Dr. James Phillips
Virginia Merrill H. Research Center/
University of Washington
Box 357923
CHDD Building, CD 176
Seattle, WA 98175-7923

Phone (206)-685-2962
bloedel@u.washington.edu

Herbert Silverstein, MD, FACS
President Silverstein Institute and Ear Research Foundation
1901 Floyd Street
Sarasota, Fla, 34239

Phone (941)-366-9222
Dr. Silverstein email/ hsilverste@aol.com

In 1978, Dr. Silverstein developed a safe approach to cut the vestibular nerve (see above surgery treatments) to prevent any damage to the brain that is located very close to the vestibular nerve.

His institute was also a pioneer in developing minimally invasive procedures that could be performed in the office. Microwick was one such a procedure and was developed so patients could treat themselves at home by placing medication in the ear canal. The Microwick absorbs the medication and carries it to the ear canal. It is used in gentamicin and steroid treatments (read treatments above)

It is a privilege to add Dr. Silverstein updated comments after reviewing the medical data pertinent to Meniere in this book.

Quoting Dr. Silverstein,

"He wholeheartedly concurs that both migraines and allergies play a part in the course of Meniere's disease. Dr. Silverstein has come up with a NEW CONCEPT which he calls "Subclinical Meniere's disease". Patients first complain of fullness and stuffiness in the ear. After other causes have been ruled out, Dr. Silverstein has found that the Microwick and dexamethasone perfusion of the inner ear for one month may abort the Meniere's disease from progressing to vertigo and hearing loss. Patients can read about this clinical study on his website under his publications. He also added that

Dr. Jay Rubinstein surgery should work. If Meniere is treated early enough in the disease with steroids there may be less patients with the vertigo."

This is an incredible research done by Dr. Silverstein. It is my wish that both the medical community as well as patients take whole advantage of it.

Dr. Timothy Hain
Northwestern University. Chicago, IL.

Chicago Dizziness and Hearing (CDH) is a private medical practice affiliated with Northwestern University. Dr. Hain specializes in diagnosis and treatment of hearing and dizziness disorders. Dr. Hain is a renowned Neurotologist voted as one of ten top physicians of Chicago. Dr. Hain is the only physician I know that administers low-dose gentamicin shots to treat bilateral Meniere's vertigo.

645 N Michigan Suite 410
Chicago, Il, USA 60611
Phone (312)-274-0197
Dr. Hain e-mail/t-hain@norhtwestern.edu

Dr. Lloyd Minor
John Hopkins University
Professor and Director of Otolaryngology
Provost Office—265 Garland Hall
3400 N. Charles Street
Baltimore, MD 21218
Phone (410) 516-8070
     (410) 614 8070

Dr. Minor e-mail/lminor@jhmi.edu

The vestibular system is responsible for sensing and controlling motion. Dr. Minor is currently researching the physiological processes that mediate the vestibular reflexes. His goal is to apply his knowledge of basic vestibular physiology to the diagnosis and treatment of balance disorders in humans. i.e. Meniere's disease.

Dr. Minor was willing at one point to treat me with intratympanic steroid shots if I could not find any other physician willing to administer the treatment in Miami. I am forever indebted to his generosity and compassion. Luckily, my local ENT, did the procedure in his office.

On July 2012, Dr. Minor was named dean of the Stanford School of Medicine. Well done, doctor!

Consult Dr. John Carey, Neurotologist/ 443 997 6467/ John Hopkins

Los Angeles House Ear Clinic and Institute
Dr. Derald Brackmann
Clinical Professor of Otolaryngology Head and Neck Surgery and Neurosurgery at the Los Angeles County USC
Medical Center.
He specializes in diseases of the ear, facial nerve, dizziness and acoustic neuromas.

Dr. Jennifer Derebery
She was elected president of the American Academy of Otolaryngology—Head and Neck Surgery for the (2003-2004) term.
She specializes in the diagnosis and treatment of allergy-related hearing loss and associated disorders.
Dr. Berebery was a co-principle investigator of a doubled-blind study on the treatment of autoimmune inner ear disease

(AIED), sponsored by the National Institutes of Health and Deafness.

House Clinic is located in Los Angeles, CA, at the corner of 3rd and Alvarado streets across from the St. Vincent's Medical Center.
Phone (213)-483-9930
www. houseearclinic.com

Emory University Department of Otolaryngology
Atlanta, GA.

Phone (404)-778-3381

Dr. Lawrence Grobman/
Otology/ Neurotology
3661 S. Miami Ave #409
Miami, Fl.
(305)-854-5971

8940 SW 88th St.
Miami, Fl.
(305)-595-6200

ESSENTIAL ADVICE FOR MENIERE

Meniere usually presents itself at middle age, but there are cases—like mine—where it may start as early as in the second decade of life.

You don't need to have all characteristic Meniere's symptoms present at the beginning of the illness to have the disease. That was my story and because I was an exception in that sense, three years elapsed after initial onset of symptoms before a final diagnosis was declared.

Don't underestimate vertigo (sensation that the room is spinning around you or you are spinning) accompanied by dizziness, loss of balance, fullness and pressure in ears, ringing (tinnitus), nausea and/ or vomiting. These are serious symptoms. Never assume that they "are just in your head" and ignore them. Seek immediate medical help, preferably from an ENT or Neurotologist specialist.

Do realize that Meniere is a chronic condition that alters your lifestyle in varying degrees. You need plenty of sleep at night. It is wise to adhere to a daily routine. Learn to slow down, take frequent breaks during the day; don't try to work at the same pace that you used to before you were diagnosed. Change line of work if necessary.

Dietary advice

Eat a low-salt diet.
Avoid caffeine and alcohol.
Have several smaller meals throughout the day instead of three square meals.
Eat healthy. Include plenty of vegetables, fresh fruits and white meats such as fish and chicken in your diet.
Avoid greasy foods. Eat your meats either grilled or baked.
Avoid refined sugar commonly present in desserts, sodas, ice-creams and candies.
Drink plenty of water, tea and natural non artificially-sweetened juices.
Take a multivitamin daily.

Lifestyle advice

When seized by an acute attack of vertigo, lie down, and take your anti-nausea and anti-vertigo medication swiftly. DON'T

MOVE YOUR HEAD. HOLD IT WITH THE PALMS OF YOUR HANDS AS TIGHLY AS YOU CAN.

You need to carry your meds wherever you go. The quicker you learn to dry swallow your meds the better for you. Water might not be always within your reach unless you carry it with you.

If vomiting is persistent, call 911 and go to a hospital immediately to avoid dehydration. Oral medications are expelled once vomiting is relentless; therefore, do not waste time. I have personally tried to ride the vomiting at home for hours. In the end, I had been in need of iv medications to arrest the crisis and possible dehydration.

DO NOT DRIVE under the spell of an attack. It might be tempting to do it when you are pressured by an important affair or errand to run but your life is more precious. If you are driving when vertigo hits you, stop the car and call a cab or 911. Do not worry about your car. You can always find somebody to help you retrieve it later.

When your Meniere is under control never venture to drive long distances by yourself. Do not drive at night either. Have someone to drive you wherever you need to go. Make sure that either a friend or a relative always know where you are.

If you use public transportation practice the same safety rules. If seized by vertigo, have somebody tell the driver you are ill and let an authority figure to help you get home or the hospital safely.

Always carry your medications and medical insurance card id with you wherever you go. Have a list at hand that specifies the current meds and doses in case you need to go to ER. Also, list all of your allergies. You might write the lists on your smartphone.

Make sure that your closest relatives and/or friends know about your medications and allergies. Inform them where you keep your list and insurance card. This is essential, especially if you live alone and/or with minor children. This precaution has been a lifesaver for me in more than an occasion.

If you ride in a car, carry your walker in the trunk always. If you walk long distances bring it with you. More than once, I have left home feeling well and I have returned leaning on my walker. Remember, Meniere is totally unpredictable.

A good night sleep is crucial to Menerians. Invest in the most comfortable mattress you can afford. If you live in a hot climate like I do, keep your room temperature cool at night. If you live in a cold climate, adjust your heater temperature to your comfort. Same advice is useful regarding bedding. I found out that I sleep my best surrounded by jersey cotton sheets and plush, soft pillows. When temperatures take a dive in the coldest months of the year, (about three or four days in Miami) I bury myself under thick down comforters and wear wide-rim plush socks to bed.

Always keep a nightlight on. If light bothers you wear an eye-mask to sleep. If you wake up dizzy you won't have trouble finding your meds since the room is softly illuminated. Besides, since Menerian's balance system is already compromised we rely on our vision to walk in the dark. Use nightlights in other important rooms of your house such as the kitchen, the bathroom and corridors. Take advantage of all the LED lighting in today's market!

Have your meds, snacks, water, walker and cell by your bedside; especially, if you live on your own. Have your closest friend or relative's phone number on speed dial.

For those times when you are too sick and your mobility is compromised, a bedside table with a microwave and a small refrigerator next to it might be a temporary solution.

Keep phone numbers handy for your doctor, hospital and someone who can take you for medical care.

If you live alone install an electronic door lock. It can be accessed with a remote control, a backlit keypad or a traditional key. If you need emergency assistance and can't walk to the door it would allow you to open it from your bed or to instruct your help how to open it. Check different models. Prices are affordable.

Exercise regularly! Even on those days when you can't go out of the house, do some light weight lifting and some basic exercises with your legs and arms to keep as fit as you can. If you feel up to it, venture outside and do some walking. On your best days, hit the gym and the pool (I don't do laps anymore out of concern for my safety, but I move my legs and arms in the water to add some resistance to my routine). Exercise can also prevent spine injuries due to lack of activity and therefore loss of muscle strength. I have had to endure a microsurgery for a lumbar hernia most likely the result of years of being confined to bed.

Resources (a list of some of my favorite stores)
Medical supply stores

iMed
www. iMed.com (wheelchairs, walkers, canes, bath seats, no rinse shampoo and conditioner)

Brylane Home
www. Brylanehome.com (bed wedge, canes, wheelchairs, wheelchair cushions, walkers, bariatric bath and shower seats,

comfort wipe with long reach bar, bath sponge with soap holder, shower sandals, hand rails, grab bars with super grips, safety 1st tub bars, shower head with hose, toilet safety frames, adjustable over bed tables, pick up and reaching tools (hand grabbers), touch neck pillow (to help immobilize neck when seized by a vertigo attack)

Brylane Home carries all personal care items for heavy set customers. Check their Plus-size living section.

Carol Wright (carries a whole array of medical products) www. Carolwright.com

Chain stores such as:
CVS, Walgreens, Bed Bath and Beyond, Wal Mart and Target sell some medical products as well. (Canes, walkers, bariatric bath seats and commodes, dry shampoo, bedside rails, grab hands, take your time to peruse over all items)

Google walkers' tennis balls and you'll find plenty of stores to purchase tennis balls to help you walker glide easily

Home Depot and Lowes (Electronic keypad deadbolt)

Tempur-Pedic beds (adjustable beds)
Their variety of ergo adjustable bases offer you virtually unlimited ergonomic positions and rejuvenating massage all controlled by a wireless remote. The ultimate sleep experience!
Visit Tempur-Pedic website.

CIL SOFL. Center for Independent Living of South Florida. Inc. www.soflacil.org
6660 Biscayne Blvd.
1st. floor
Miami, Fl. 33138
305 751 8025

The Center for Independent Living of South Florida offers services free of charge to persons with disabilities. They help people with physical, sensory (deafness and blindness), mental or emotional conditions regardless of age or income. Their Deaf Center lends phone equipment for hard of hearing, deaf, deaf/blind with volume/tone control panels, TTY's (Telecommunication device for the deaf) and increased volume/visual phone signals on a long term basis at no charge to the consumer. I borrowed my amplified telephone from them. It is a worthy piece of equipment. It allows me to communicate with people much better than before. All you need is a form, the FTRI (Florida Telecommunications Relay, Inc.) application, signed by your doctor or audiologist to obtain one.

If you are not a Florida resident, find out if your state has a telephone loan equipment program. Most sates do.

Important Organizations for the Hearing Impaired and Balance Disorders

Hearing Loss Association of America

National Association of the Deaf

The Deaf Service Center Association Inc.

Meniere's Disease Information Center

www.MenieresInfo.com (Check all current Meniere Clinical Trials to see if you can participate; they are free. All sorts of insightful information about Meniere)

www.Menieres.org (Information and support for all Menierians and their relatives. Includes message boards, chat rooms, journal entries)

Depression

Seek medical help.

Take your medications religiously.

Get involved in psychotherapy.

Exercise regularly. Even a short walk outside of your home is helpful.

Seek outside help around the house if needed.

Do not shut out your friends.

Avoid sad news.

Get rid of negative, poisoning influences in your life.

Forgive and let God do justice for you.

Watch funny movies and TV programs.

Listen to joyful, uplifting or relaxing music depending on your mood. Music has magic, soothing powers!

Surround yourself by calming scents. Sprinkle lavender on your linens. Immerse yourself in a scented bubble bath. Light-up some vanilla or other fragrant pleasant candle while listening to some relaxing music. Drink some peppermint tea or a warm cup of milk. In my own experience, a warm shower followed by a warm glass of milk and my meds right before bedtime always soothe my nerves, and ensue the most restful night!

Read and research books and articles about your condition.

Indispensable books to cope with Depression, Anxiety and Stress and Other Mental Conditions

The Dance of Anger: A Woman's Guide to Changing the Pattern of Intimate Relationships for Women by Harriet Lerner.

Anxiety and stress stems from high expectations, and frustrations when those expectations are not met. This book is highly recommended to repair relationships.

Living the Truth by Dr. Kieth Ablow. Learn the whys, whats, wheres and how we got to the messes we are. Learn how to identify and break learned unhealthy mental behaviors turning them into a new future.

Overcoming Depression One Step at a Time by Michael Addis and Christopher Martell

This workbook is filled of exercises and ideas to inspire you with feelings of pleasure as powerful antidotes against depression.

Feel the Fear and . . . Do it Anyway. Dynamic techniques for turning fear, indecision, and anger into power, action and love by Susan Jeffers.

Psychologist Jeffers discusses the crippling effects of fear in her own life and how she formulated a course of action to conquer it.

Get It Done When You're Depressed. 50 Strategies for Keeping Your Life on Track by Julie Fast John D. Preston, Psy.D.

In this book readers will learn how to prepare themselves mentally for working while being depressed, how to structure their days and how to prevent depression.

The Other Side of Me. Autobiography by Sidney Sheldon, producer and writer of famous television shows such as I Dream of Jeannie and Hart to Hart and victim of Bipolar Disorder.

Take Charge of Bipolar: A 4 Step Plan for You and Your Loved Ones to Manage the Illness and Create Stability By Julie Fast and John Preston.

Julie Fast is the founder of Bipolar Happens, a popular online resource. She was diagnosed at age 31 and is now a recognized expert in the field. John Preston is a neuropsychologist specializing in Bipolar Disorder.

Beyond the Blues: A Workbook to Help Teens Overcome Depression by Lisa Schab, LCSW.

This workbook offers exercises to help teenagers make small changes in their lives to cope with sad feelings, help them to make new friends and deal with conflicts.

When Nothing Matters Anymore: A Survival Guide for Depressed Teens. By Beverly Cobain nurse and cousin of Kurt Cobain, deceased lead singer and guitarist of musical group Nirvana and victim of Bipolar Disorder and Depression.

Beyond the Blues: A Guide to Understanding and Treating Prenatal and Postpartum Depression. By Shoshanna S. Bennett, PhD. and Pec Indman, Ed.D.

The book contains current information about risks factors, diagnosis and treatment of mood disorders in pregnancy and postpartum. This book is being used by the US Navy, New York State Health Department, the International Childbirth Education organization and many other organizations.

What To Say To When You Talk to Yourself by Shad Helmstetter, Ph.D.

Most of us talk to ourselves all day long without even realizing it! The problem is we hammer our brains with bitter criticism and negative thoughts. This book would teach you how to talk to yourself in new, positive, and constructive ways. Awesome!

The Gift: The 12 Greatest Tools of Personal Growth and How to Put Them into Practice by Shad Helmstetter.

The Gift is the inspiring story of women and men who are changing their lives—by helping others change theirs.

Read uplifting books.
These are some of my favorites

The Bible. The books of Psalms and Ecclesiastes are my favorites from the Old Testament

The New Testament

Chicken Soup for Unsinkable Souls
Chicken Soup for the Woman's Soul
A Second Chicken Soup for the Woman's Soul
Chicken Soup Christmas Stories all of them by Jack Canfield and Mark Hansen

Your Best Life Now and Become a Better You:7 Steps to Living at your Full Potential by Pastor Joel Osteen

Mother Angelica, The Remarkable Story of a Nun, Her Nerve and a Network of Miracles by Raymond Arroyo.

Mother Angelica's unique witty humor and tenacity to build the multinational catholic network EWTN will bring tears of joy and admiration to your heart.

Keep Climbing by Sean Swarmer, the striking story of a teenager who was diagnosed with two types of terminal cancers and he survived both! He has dedicated his life after his miraculous remission's to climb the tallest mountains of the world including Mt. Everest; a true inspirational story you don't want to miss!

Unmeasured Strength by Lauren Manning.

On September 11, 2001 Lauren's body was engulfed by a wall of flame at the Trade World Center that burned more than 80 percent of her body. This is the riveting story of Lauren's ten-year miraculous journey of survival and reconstruction of her precious life and that of her family and the thousands of 9/11 attacks survivor victims. Her story has been on The Oprah Winfrey show, NBC's Today and many other media outlets.

He is Gone You are Back by Kerika Fields. A true gem for women who are going through a breakup and need all the cheerful, wise advice they can get to avoid falling into the trap of depression; it is full of great tips for all the marvelous ladies out there struggling with depression whatever the cause might be. You'll really enjoy Kerika's savvy hints and who knows the book might come handy for one of your friends or yourself if you are experiencing some heartache of your own.

O's Big Book of Happiness. The Best of Oprah magazine.
A wonderful recompilation of the best Oprah's magazine articles in all areas of our lives, including precious advice for mental health.

Hilarious books to get you laughing and engaged from beginning to end.

Why My Third Husband Will be a Dog and My Nest Isn't Empty, It Just Has More Closet Space by Lisa Scottoline.

Shopaholic series by Sophie Kinsella.

Remember you can check out books from your local library. They are free!
With the meteoric rise of tablets, smartphones and online retailers such as Amazon, Kindle and Nook, it is easier than ever to access books and all sort of medical information. You can even borrow e-books from your library nowadays.

My favorite movies to tickle your funny bone
To be watched with young kids (including the one inside you)

Mulan,
The Emperors's New Groove
Aristocats
The Little Mermaid
Sleeping Beauty

Cinderella
Madagascar series
Pirates of the Caribbean series
The Princess Bride
Cool Runnings
The Princess Diary I & II
The Sound Of Music
Toy Story
Ratatouille

For the adults

Ocean's 11, 12, & 13 (Brad Pitt, George Clooney, Julia Roberts)
Miss Congeniality I & II (Sandra Bullock)
Date Night
Sister Act I & II (Whoopi Goldberg)
Jumping Jack Flash (Whoopi Goldberg)
Young Frankenstein directed by Mel Brooks (Gene Wilder)
Haunted Honeymoon (Gene Wilder)
Mamma Mia (Meryl Streep) Abba's Music
Beauty Shop (Queen Latifah)
Last Holiday (Queen Latifah)
Enchanted
America's Sweethearts (Julia Roberts, Billy Crystal, Zeta Jones)
The Pink Panther series (Peter Sellers)
Confessions of a Shopaholic
The Devil Wears Prada
Dumb and Dumber
The 40-Year-Old Virgin
Anchorman: The Legend of Ron Burg
Billy Madison
Borat

Pray, meditate and get closer to God; every single day!
Infallible advice! Get out of your shell and help others!
My mantra for depression is "Ora et Labora". Pray and Work.
A crafty project of your liking and charity works can do wonders to
brighten up your days!

Depression resources for advocacy, referrals and immediate help.

NAMI. The National Alliance on Mental Illness is the nation's
largest grassroots mental health organization dedicated to build
better lives for millions of Americans affected by mental illness.
NAMI focuses on support, education, research and advocacy to
help individuals and families affected by mental illness.

Information Helpline
1-800-950-NAMI (6264)
Spanish
1-703-524-760
info@nami.org

PAIMI. Protection and Advocacy for Individuals with Mental Illness.

The purposes of PAIMI are:

To protect and advocate the rights of individuals with mental illness.
To investigate incidents of abuse or neglect of individuals with
    mental illness.

1-800-245-4743
advocate@disabiltyrightsmt.org

NIMH. National Institute of Mental Health
www.nimh.nih.gov
866 615 6464

National Suicide Prevention Organization
www.spr.org
1-800-273-TALK
8255

Depression and Bipolar Support Alliance
www.dbsalliance.org
800 826 3632

Teen depression
www.helpguide.org/mental/depression_teen.htm

Post-Partum Depression
www.womenshealth.gov
800 994 9662

Migraine headaches.

Consult a neurologist for both preventive and pain medications. Imitrex coupled with two Advil is the most reliable pain relief. Make sure you take your meds as directed by your doctor!

Nowadays, there are a myriad of medications in the same medicine family as Imitrex (Tryptans) that are also used to treat migraines.

Preventive medications include some anti-depressants and medicines like Topamax. They are all have been used with success to reduce the number of attacks. Remember, DO NOT TAKE any medicine without consulting with a specialist first!

Take your preventive medication as indicated. Take your pain medication as soon as pain starts. A slight delay can amount to a big difference in the prompt abatement of your pain.

Apply an ice bag and/ or small ice-cold towels to dull pain.

Lie down, draw the curtains, turn off lights and shield from all noise if you can. Wear an eye mask.

Have somebody to massage your affected area. If nobody is available, massage your head yourself.

Make a fist and apply pressure to affected area for as long as you need to stop the blood flow in the throbbing area. I have tried this remedy for hours at a time when nothing else seemed to work and it has stopped the pain altogether after a while (I always take my medication first; applying pressure is an additional step).

Eat four to six small balanced meals throughout the day instead of three.

Avoid refined sugars!

Your beauty sleep is of an essence to avoid a migraine.

Hunger and lack of sleep are main triggers. So is stress.

Relax and meditate every day.

For the most hopeless chronic patients there is a surgery, neurostimulation therapy procedure. It relies in the concept that instead of taking pills to regulate severe discomfort you could use stimulation to override pain signals to the brain. The procedure involves implanting tiny, mildly vibrating wires under the skin at the site of pain; the electrical impulses block the pain signals from reaching the brain. If your life has been totally disrupted by migraines and eliminating all refined carbs from your diet do not improve your condition this surgery might be your life saver.

Migraines are very stubborn. Sometimes, the attacks might be present for weeks. Do not wait more than 24 hours if your pain persists and your regular medications do not seem to help. Visit your doctor or a hospital ER.

In the span of almost twenty years I have only had a migraine attack severe enough that lasted for over two weeks. My neurologist prescribed a "Special cocktail" of medications to arrest the pain and stop the cycle. The cocktail consisted of a prescription-strength NSAID, Imitrex, Valium, Benadryl and Zofran. This meds were to be taken for not longer than 3 days under the strict supervision of my clinician. Yes, they knocked me out, completely; but after 24 hours the migraine was gone.

LATEST NEWS FOR MIGRAINES

AS OF YEAR 2010, THE FDA HAS APPROVED A BOTOX PROCEDURE TO TREAT CHRONIC MIGRAINES THAT LAST MORE THAN FIFTEEN DAYS PER MONTH

THE NEW TREATMENT CONSISTS OF 31 BOTOX SHOTS AROUND THE EYES, TEMPLES, BACK OF THE HEAD, AND NECK.

THE EFFECT MIGHT LAST UP TO THREE MONTHS. MOST INSURANCE COMPANIES ARE COVERING THIS NEW PROCEDURE

CONSULT YOUR PHYSICIAN. DO NOT SUFFER. DO NOT TAKE ANY MEDICATIONS WITHOUT PROPER DOCTOR RECOMMENDATTION.

Menopause

The most comprehensive book about menopause I have ever read is *The Wisdom of Menopause* by Dr. Christiane Northrop.

Klippel-Treanaunay Syndrome (KTS).

Consult a vascular specialist. Wear compression stockings. Elevate your affected limb at regular intervals. Avoid standing up or walking for long periods of time. Swimming and bicycling are the best exercises for KTS patients.

National Organization for Rare Disorders (NORD)
www.rarediseases.org
203-744-0100

Vascular Birthmarks Foundation
www.birthmark.org
877-823-4646

TOP FIVE ADVICES FOR MENIERE, MIGRAINES, DEPRESSION AND ALL CHRONIC ILLNESSES.

1. Be your own advocate. If you are not satisfied with the answers you are getting, keep searching until you find the doctor with the right answer. It may take time and effort but somehow, somewhere there is a specialist who will be able to help you. Use the internet to your advantage in your quest!
2. Do not delay to seek professional help.
3. Avoid stress. It is imperative.
4. Rest as much as you can and need. Our bodies need enough hours of sleep when we are healthy to function properly, indispensable when we are sick.
5. Keep a positive outlook. Surround yourself by positive people who love you. Love is powerful. In many instances, we do not heal fast enough because we are not truly loved, because of all of the losses in our lives. If you do not have a close knit family to support you, join a group, whether is at your place of worship, a charity group or a group with a same interest as you have. Do not forget to return love to those who need it.